The Complete Guide to Oblique

Vertical Ab Workout

Mastering Technique, Variations, and Programming

Helen Talbott

Disclaimer

The information contained in this publication is for informational purposes only and is not intended to be a substitute for professional medical advice, diagnosis, or treatment. Always consult with a healthcare professional before starting any new exercise program, especially if you have any pre-existing medical conditions, injuries, or concerns. The author and publisher disclaim any and all liability for any injury or health problems that may arise from the use of the information contained herein.

Table of contents

Disclaimer
The Enemy in the Mirror
About the author
Introduction
Decoding Your Core - A Map to V abs Mastery
Conquering or Conceding? Who Should (and Shouldn't) Do Oblique V abs
Conquering or Conceding? Who Should (and Shouldn't) Do Oblique V abs
Beyond Aesthetics - Unveiling the Hidden Powers of Oblique V abs
Unlocking the V abs - Mastering the Basic Technique
Variations of the Oblique V abs
Designing an Oblique V abs Training Program
Supersets, drop sets, and other advanced training methods
Bonus Materials
Conclusion
Requesting a Review

The Enemy in the Mirror

My reflection mocked me in the gym mirror. My stomach, round and soft, seemed to mock the chiseled bodies surrounding me. "Never gonna happen," it whispered. V abs, the bane of my existence, stared back from the workout board, a smirking challenge. I'd always hated them, a flailing mess of limbs yearning for the sweet release of the floor.

One day, exhaustion gnawed at me more than usual. Defeated, I sat down, ready to quit. A voice, gruff but kind, startled me. It was Coach Mike, a pillar of strength in the gym. "Struggling with V abs?" he chuckled, not unkindly. I mumbled a sheepish yes.

"They're tough," he conceded, "but worth it. Want a different approach?" I nodded, surprised. He didn't bombard me with perfect form or impossible sets. Instead, he broke down the movement, emphasizing slow, controlled reps, engaging my core rather than flinging myself around.

That day, I managed three shaky V abs. Three! Pathetic, but Coach Mike cheered me on. He became my V abs guru, not pushing, but encouraging, celebrating every victory, no matter how small. Slowly, the V abs monster became less intimidating. My core woke up, muscles screaming but learning.

Weeks turned into months. The mirror started showing a different story. Not washboard abs overnight, but definition peeking through, a tightening where flab once lived. The V abs, once my nemesis, became a source of pride. I craved the burn, the feeling of strength building with each controlled rep.

But it wasn't just physical. Each conquered V abs chipped away at self-doubt. With each set, I pushed past perceived limitations, proving to myself I could achieve what I thought impossible. The gym became a metaphor for life, the V abs a symbol of resilience.

Today, when I see someone struggling with V abs, I remember my journey. I share Coach

Mike's wisdom, a testament to the power of small wins and unwavering belief. And when I look in the mirror, I see not just a stronger core, but a reflection of determination, the woman who conquered the V abs and, in doing so, conquered a bit of herself.

Sweat plastered itself to my forehead, stinging my eyes in a mocking welcome to the gym. Today, as always, the enemy awaited in the form of the V abs board. Five perfect silhouettes arched impossibly upwards, their sculpted abs seeming to taunt my own round, jiggly stomach. Every time I saw them, a voice whispered in my head, "Never gonna happen."

About the author

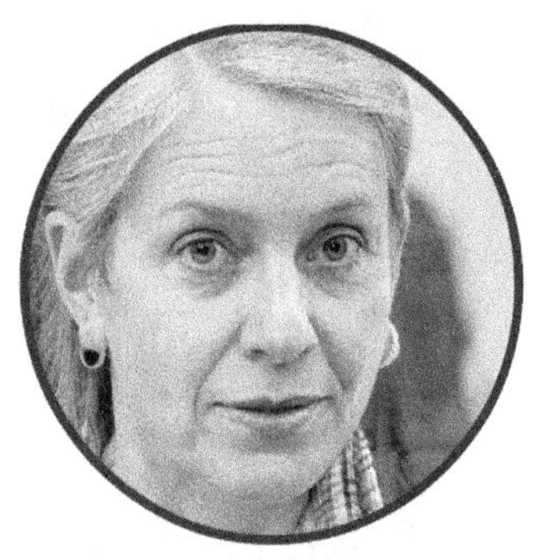

As Helen Talbott, I invite you to embark on a journey to conquer the elusive oblique V abs. With over 8 years of experience in fitness and a passion for movement, I've meticulously crafted this guide to empower you to master this core-crushing exercise.

My first encounter with the V abs was one of pure intimidation. It was during a group fitness class, and the instructor casually announced we'd be moving on to "V abs." Everyone around me seemed unfazed, but my core instantly lurched into panic mode. Visions of flopping helplessly on the mat like a fish out of water flooded my mind.

Determined not to wimp out, I cautiously lowered myself onto the mat. The first attempt was...rough. My upper body barely left the ground, and my lower back screamed in protest.

Frustration gnawed at me. Was I really that inflexible? That weak?

The instructor, sensing my struggle, offered some pointers. She emphasized keeping my core engaged, drawing my belly button towards my spine, and using controlled movements rather than flinging myself up. With trepidation, I tried again.

This time, something shifted. I could feel my core muscles working, pulling me upwards like a marionette controlled by invisible strings. Slowly, shakily, I managed to lift my torso off the mat, forming a graceful V with my body. It wasn't perfcct, but it was a V!

Exhilaration washed over me. Each subsequent repetition felt a little smoother, a little stronger. By the end of the set, I wasn't just completing the reps, I was almost enjoying them. This exercise that had initially petrified me was starting to feel empowering.

Over the weeks, my V abs journey continued. Some days were better than others. There were moments of doubt, days when my core felt like a bowl of overcooked spaghetti. But with each practice session, I could see (and feel) progress. My movements became more fluid, my core grew stronger, and the initial fear was replaced by a sense of accomplishment.

Now, the V abs is no longer a source of intimidation, but a badge of honor. It's a reminder of how far I've come, of the strength I never knew I possessed. It's a test of not just my physical capabilities, but also my mental resolve. And each time I conquer that "V," it's a victory not just over the exercise, but over self-doubt.

So, if you're hesitant to try the V abs, I encourage you to take the plunge. It might be challenging, it might be humbling, but it could also be the start of a rewarding journey towards a stronger, more confident you. Remember, progress over perfection, and every V, imperfect as it may be, is a step towards mastery.

Through trial and error, I discovered the key nuances that unlock their full potential. This guide is the culmination of that journey, filled with insights gleaned from countless hours of practice and a deep understanding of biomechanics.

Why Choose Helen Talbott as Your Guide?

- **Expertise:** My background allows me to provide a comprehensive understanding of the exercise, ensuring you approach it with both safety and effectiveness.
- **Passion:** My enthusiasm for oblique V abs is contagious, and I'm committed to helping you achieve your fitness goals with this exercise.
- **Clarity:** I explain complex concepts in a clear, concise, and engaging manner, making the guide accessible to all fitness levels.
- **Results-Oriented:** My focus is on providing practical and actionable steps that deliver tangible results.

What You'll Find in The Complete Guide to Oblique V abs:

- **Mastering the Technique:** Break down the movement step-by-step, ensuring perfect form and maximum activation of your obliques.
- **Unleashing Variations:** Explore a diverse range of oblique V abs variations to keep your workouts fresh and challenging.
- **Programming for Progress:** Discover effective workout routines that fit your fitness level and goals, helping you see consistent progress.
- **Troubleshooting Common Mistakes:** Learn how to avoid common pitfalls and ensure you're getting the most out of each rep.
- **Science-Backed Insights:** Gain a deeper understanding of the exercise's benefits and the science behind its effectiveness.

Join me, Helen Talbott, on this exciting journey to oblique V abs mastery. Let's

unlock your core potential and achieve the sculpted physique you desire!

Introduction

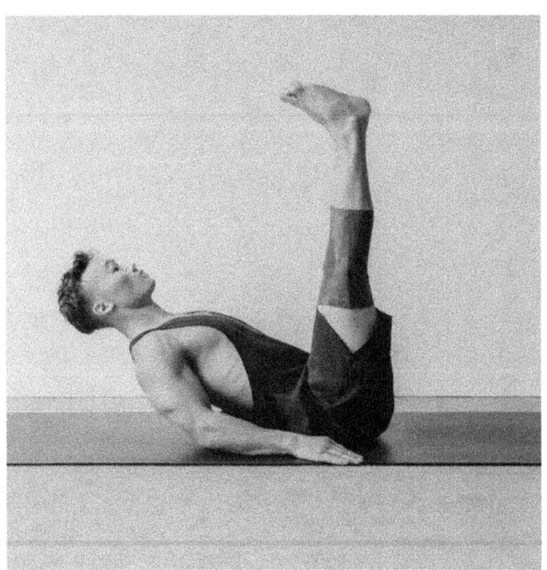

Remember the enemy in the mirror? Well, buckle up, because it's time to introduce you to its nemesis: the **oblique V abs**. It may look intimidating, a contortionist's dream come true, but this exercise holds the key to unlocking sculpted abs, a stronger core, and a newfound confidence.

But before we launch into conquering V abs like fearless warriors, let's demystify the beast. Unlike regular crunches that target your rectus abdominis (the "six-pack" muscle), oblique V abs focus on your **obliques**, the diagonally running muscles along your sides. These unsung heroes play a crucial role in:

- **Rotational power:** Whether you're throwing a punch, swinging a tennis racket, or twisting to avoid a rogue toddler, strong obliques provide the stability and power needed for rotational movements.
- **Core stability:** Think of your core as your body's powerhouse. Strong obliques contribute to a rock-solid midsection, essential for good posture, preventing back pain, and improving overall athletic performance.
- **Sculpting definition:** Want that coveted hourglass figure or V-shaped torso? Oblique V abs help carve definition not just in your abs, but also in your sides,

creating a more aesthetically pleasing silhouette.

Now, the "V" in V abs isn't just for show. This exercise gets its name from the V-shaped position your body forms as you lift your torso and legs off the ground simultaneously. It might seem complex initially, but fret not, for we'll break down the mechanics and variations in the next chapter.

Remember, the transformation journey starts with a single step. So, cast aside your fear of the V abs monster, embrace the challenge, and get ready to unleash your inner core ninja! After all, conquering this exercise isn't just about sculpted abs, it's about proving to yourself that you can achieve anything you set your mind to. So, are you ready to join the V abs revolution?

Chapter 1

Decoding Your Core - A Map to V abs Mastery

Before we delve into the mechanics of the V abs, let's take a quick detour to understand the key players involved: your core muscles. Think of them as your body's internal power station, responsible for stability, posture, and movement. But within this power station, specific muscles shine when it comes to V abs – the **obliques**.

Meet the Obliques:

- **Internal Obliques:** These deep-seated muscles run diagonally from your lower ribs to your pelvis, pulling your torso downwards and inwards. Imagine them like internal seatbelts, stabilizing your spine during twists and rotations.
- **External Obliques:** These surface-level muscles form the V-shape we associate with V abs. They extend from your ribs

down to your pelvis and pubic bone, responsible for rotating your torso and drawing your belly button inwards.

These two oblique heroes work together during V abs, with the internal obliques initiating the movement and the external obliques providing power and control. But remember, your core is more than just the obliques. Other players like the **rectus abdominis** (your "six-pack") and **transverse abdominis** (your deep core corset) also contribute to core stability and support the V abs movement.

Understanding the Connection:

Visualize your core muscles like interconnected threads forming a supportive web around your spine and pelvis. When you engage your obliques in a V abs, you're not just working isolated muscles; you're activating this entire network, leading to improved core strength, stability, and coordination.

Think of it like building a house of cards. Strong individual cards (muscles) are crucial, but it's the interconnectedness that creates a stable structure (your core). V abs help strengthen these connections, leading to a more robust and functional core.

Beyond the Obliques:

While the obliques take center stage during V abs, remember that core training is holistic. Don't neglect other core muscles like the rectus abdominis and transverse abdominis. Performing a variety of core exercises alongside V abs ensures a well-rounded and balanced core development.

Remember, knowledge is power! Understanding the anatomy of your core and how the obliques function in V abs will help you approach the exercise with more focus and control. Now, armed with this newfound knowledge, let's tackle the mechanics of the V abs in the next chapter!

Chapter 2

Conquering or Conceding? Who Should (and Shouldn't) Do Oblique V abs

The allure of sculpted abs and a stronger core is undeniable, but not every exercise fits everyone. So, before you dive headfirst into the world of V abs, let's explore who can benefit from this exercise and who might need to consider alternative approaches.

The V abs Fan Club:

- **Fitness enthusiasts:** Whether you're a seasoned athlete or a fitness newbie, oblique V abs can add variety and challenge to your core routine, improving strength, stability, and rotational power.
- **Those seeking sculpted abs:** Yes, V abs are known for targeting the obliques, contributing to that coveted V-shaped torso and overall core definition.

- **People seeking improved core stability:** Strong obliques contribute to a stable core, essential for good posture, preventing back pain, and enhancing athletic performance.
- **Those recovering from injuries (with caution):** Under the guidance of a healthcare professional, modified V abs can be incorporated into post-rehabilitation programs to strengthen core muscles weakened by injury.

The "Proceed with Caution" Crew:

- **Individuals with pre-existing back problems:** If you have lower back pain, disc issues, or other spinal conditions, consult your doctor before attempting V abs. Improper form can exacerbate these issues.
- **Pregnant women:** While core engagement is important during pregnancy, V abs may put undue strain on your abdominal muscles and ligaments.

Opt for modified core exercises suitable for pregnancy.

- **Those with limited flexibility:** If you struggle with basic core exercises like crunches due to tightness in your hamstrings or hip flexors, V abs might be too challenging at the moment. Focus on improving flexibility and core strength with easier exercises first.
- **Beginner with poor form:** It's crucial to master proper form before diving into V abs. Attempting them with poor technique can lead to injury. Consider seeking guidance from a certified trainer or physical therapist to learn the correct form.

Remember, listening to your body is paramount. If you experience any pain or discomfort during V abs, stop immediately and consult a healthcare professional before continuing.

Alternative Options:

Don't despair if V abs aren't for you! Plenty of other exercises effectively target your core and obliques. Consider planks, side planks, Russian twists, or bicycle crunches for similar benefits.

The key is finding exercises that fit your fitness level, limitations, and goals. With the right approach and alternative options, everyone can build a strong and functional core, sculpted abs or not.

So, are you ready to join the V abs revolution? If yes, proceed with caution and proper guidance. If not, remember, there are other paths to core strength and a healthy you!

Chapter 3

Beyond Aesthetics - Unveiling the Hidden Powers of Oblique V abs

Sure, V abs might pique your interest for sculpted abs, but their benefits extend far beyond aesthetics. So, buckle up as we delve into the hidden powers of this exercise, transforming your perception from "crunch alternative" to "core powerhouse".

Unleashing Core Strength:

- **Core Stability Powerhouse:** Forget just "six-pack abs". V abs engage your entire core, including the often-neglected obliques. This translates to a rock-solid midsection, crucial for good posture, preventing back pain, and excelling in various sports.
- **Rotational Power Unleashed:** Imagine throwing a punch, swinging a racket, or

twisting to avoid a flying toy. Strong obliques, honed by V abs, provide the stability and power needed for these rotational movements, boosting your athletic performance.
- **Improved Functional Movement:** Daily activities like bending, lifting, and reaching involve core engagement. V abs enhance core strength and stability, making these everyday movements smoother and more efficient.

Beyond the Physical:

- **Confidence Boost:** Conquering the V abs challenge isn't just about physical gains. It's a testament to your willpower and discipline, boosting your confidence and self-belief in both fitness and other areas of life.
- **Stress Buster:** Feeling overwhelmed? V abs can be a powerful stress reliever. The focused movement and exertion act as a release valve, leaving you feeling invigorated and mentally sharper.

- **Better Balance:** Strong obliques contribute to overall balance and coordination, reducing your risk of falls and injuries, especially as you age.

Remember, consistency is key! Regular V abs practice unlocks these benefits progressively. Start slow, master the form, and gradually increase the repetitions and sets as your strength improves.

But wait, there's more! V abs offer flexibility too. The dynamic movement stretches your hamstrings and hip flexors, improving your overall range of motion and preventing stiffness.

A Word of Caution:

While V abs are fantastic, improper form can lead to injury. Ensure you understand the correct technique and listen to your body. If you experience pain, stop immediately and consult a healthcare professional.

In the next chapter, we'll delve into the magical world of V abs variations, ensuring you have the perfect exercise to fit your fitness level and goals. So, get ready to unlock the full potential of V abs and unleash your inner core ninja!

Chapter 4

Unlocking the V abs - Mastering the Basic Technique

Now that you're armed with the knowledge of V abs benefits and limitations, it's time to unveil the secret weapon – **mastering the basic V abs technique**. Remember, proper form is paramount for maximizing benefits and minimizing injury risk. So, grab your mat and prepare to conquer this core challenge!

Step-by-Step Guide:

1. **Prepare for liftoff:** Lie on your side with legs extended and stacked on top of each other. Place your bottom arm flat on the mat for support and rest your top arm behind your head with your elbow bent. Engage your core by drawing your belly button inwards.
2. **Initiate the V:** Inhale as you simultaneously lift your torso and legs off

the ground. Aim for a diagonal movement, forming a V shape with your body. Imagine your chest reaching towards your hip while your legs extend straight. Keep your core engaged throughout the movement.

3. **Reach and squeeze:** At the peak of the V, hold for a second and squeeze your obliques, feeling the contraction on your sides. Don't yank your neck with your hand; keep your head in line with your spine.

4. **Controlled descent:** Exhale as you slowly lower your torso and legs back down to the starting position, maintaining core engagement throughout. Don't let your body flop onto the mat. Control the descent!

5. **Repeat and conquer:** This is one rep. Aim for 8-12 repetitions on each side for starters, gradually increasing reps and sets as you get stronger. Remember, quality over quantity!

Pro Tips for Perfect Form:

- **Focus on core engagement:** It's not just about lifting your body; think about actively drawing your belly button inwards throughout the movement.
- **Maintain a straight back:** Avoid arching your back; keep it flat and engaged.
- **Don't strain your neck:** Keep your chin slightly tucked and avoid pulling your head up with your hands.
- **Breathe!** Inhale during the descent and exhale during the V abs.
- **Slow and controlled:** Don't rush the movement. Focus on smooth, controlled reps for optimal results.

Common Mistakes to Avoid:

- **Swinging your body:** The movement should be controlled and powered by your core, not momentum.
- **Lifting your legs too high:** Focus on forming a diagonal V-shape, not raising your legs straight up.

- **Ignoring your core:** Remember, it's all about engaging your core muscles, not just using your arms to lift yourself.
- **Pushing your limits:** Start slow and gradually increase the difficulty as you progress. Don't push yourself to pain or discomfort.

Remember, mastering the basic V abs takes practice. Be patient, focus on form, and celebrate every conquered rep. In the next chapter, we'll explore exciting variations to add spice to your V abs routine and keep your core challenged. Get ready to take your training to the next level!

Step-by-Step Breakdown of the Oblique V abs
with Visual Cues:

Preparation:

1. **Lie on your side:** Start by lying on one
   side with your legs extended and stacked
   on top of each other. Ensure your body
   forms a straight line from head to toe.
2. **Support and engagement:** Place your
   bottom arm flat on the mat for support and
   prop your top arm behind your head with
   your elbow bent at a 90-degree angle.
   Engage your core by drawing your belly
   button inwards towards your spine.
   Imagine zipping up an imaginary corset
   around your midsection.

The V abs:

1. **Initiate the lift:** Inhale as you
   simultaneously lift your upper torso and
   legs off the ground. Think about initiating
   the movement from your core, not
   throwing yourself up with your arms.

2. **Form the V:** Aim for a diagonal movement, forming a V shape with your body. Imagine your chest reaching towards the opposite hip while your legs extend straight out, maintaining a slight bend in your knees for safety.
3. **Peak and squeeze:** Hold this V-shaped position for a second at the top. Squeeze your obliques, feeling the contraction on the sides of your torso. Keep your core engaged and avoid arching your back.
4. **Controlled descent:** Exhale as you slowly lower your torso and legs back down to the starting position in a controlled manner. Resist the urge to flop onto the mat; maintain core engagement throughout.

Key Points:

- **Focus on core:** Remember, this is a core exercise, not a neck or arm exercise. Focus on engaging your core throughout the movement, drawing your belly button inwards and keeping your back flat.

- **Controlled movement:** Avoid jerky movements. Both the ascent and descent should be smooth and controlled.
- **Breathe:** Inhale as you descend and exhale as you lift. Proper breathing helps maintain core stability and prevents dizziness.
- **Listen to your body:** Start slow and gradually increase reps and sets as you get stronger. Don't push yourself to pain or discomfort.

Visual Cues:

- Imagine your body forming a perfect diagonal V from head to toe at the peak of the movement.
- Think about squeezing a grapefruit between your obliques at the top hold.
- Visualize lowering yourself down as if you're slowly being lowered by a string attached to your chest.

Remember: Mastering the V abs takes practice and patience. Focus on proper form, celebrate your progress, and enjoy the journey towards a stronger and more sculpted core!

Bonus Tip: For an added challenge, try placing a light weight (like a water bottle) behind your head at the top of the V abs. Remember to prioritize form over weight and start light.

Conquering the V abs: Avoiding Common Mistakes for Optimal Results

Mastering the V abs requires more than just lifting yourself off the ground. Proper form is crucial for maximizing benefits and minimizing the risk of injury. Let's dive into some common mistakes and how to avoid them:

Mistake 1: Swinging your body

Symptom: You use momentum to fling yourself up instead of engaging your core.

Fix: Focus on initiating the movement from your core, feeling a deep contraction with each rep. Imagine pulling your belly button towards your spine as you lift. Slow down the movement and prioritize control over speed.

Mistake 2: Lifting your legs too high

Symptom: Your legs reach straight up in the air, forming an L shape instead of a V.

Fix: Aim for a diagonal movement where your chest reaches towards your opposite hip and your legs extend out and slightly down, forming a V shape. This engages your obliques more effectively.

Mistake 3: Ignoring your core

Symptom: You rely on your arms or neck to lift yourself, neglecting core engagement.

Fix: Remember, the V abs is all about your core! Draw your belly button inwards throughout the movement and focus on feeling the contraction in your obliques. Think about squeezing an imaginary grapefruit between your sides at the peak of the V.

Mistake 4: Pushing your limits

Symptom: You try too many reps or weights too soon, leading to fatigue, form breakdown, or injury.

Fix: Start slow and gradually increase the difficulty as you get stronger. Focus on quality over quantity and prioritize perfect form over additional reps or weight. Don't be afraid to modify the exercise if needed.

Mistake 5: Arching your back

Symptom: Your lower back hyperextends during the movement, putting strain on your spine.

Fix: Maintain a flat back throughout the exercise. Engage your core muscles to keep your spine neutral and avoid arching your lower back. Imagine pressing your lower back into the mat as you lift.

Mistake 6: Holding your breath

Symptom: You forget to breathe during the reps, limiting oxygen flow and causing dizziness.

Fix: Establish a consistent breathing pattern. Inhale as you lower yourself down and exhale as you lift your torso and legs. Proper breathing helps maintain core stability and prevents lightheadedness.

Mistake 7: Rushing the movement

Symptom: You perform jerky reps with poor control, increasing the risk of injury.

Fix: Slow down and focus on smooth, controlled movements. Feel each muscle activation throughout the V abs, from the initiation to the descent. Imagine you're performing the exercise underwater, requiring deliberate and controlled movements.

Remember: Everyone learns at their own pace. Be patient with yourself, focus on the journey, and celebrate every conquered rep with proper form. By avoiding these common mistakes, you'll be well on your way to mastering the V abs and unlocking its amazing benefits for a stronger, sculpted core!

Conquering the V abs Mountain: Progressions for Beginner Climbers

The V abs might seem like a summit reserved for seasoned core ninjas, but fear not, aspiring climbers! With the right progressions, even beginners can scale this core challenge and reap its benefits. Here's your roadmap to V abs mastery:

Step 1: Build the Foundation:

Before attempting full V abs, ensure your core has the basic strength and stability needed. Start with these foundational exercises:

- **Plank:** This isometric exercise engages your entire core, building overall strength and endurance. Aim for 3 sets of 30-second holds.

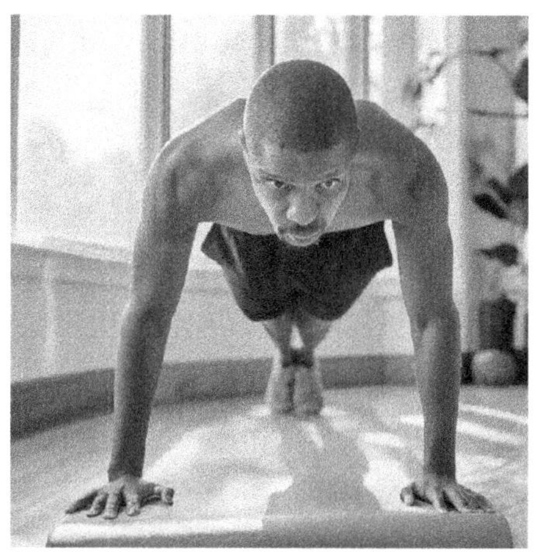

- **Bird-dog:** This exercise challenges core stability and coordination. Start on all fours, alternate extending one arm and the opposite leg, maintaining a flat back. Do 3 sets of 10 reps per side.
- **Dead bug:** Lying on your back with knees bent and feet flat, slowly lower one leg towards the ground while keeping your lower back pressed into the mat. Repeat with the other leg. Do 3 sets of 10 reps per side.

Step 2: Prepare for Takeoff:

Once you've established a solid foundation, it's time to practice the key components of the V abs:

- **Side plank:** Hold a side plank on each side for 3 sets of 30 seconds, engaging your obliques and core to stay stable.
- **Knee-up V abs:** Lie on your side, engage your core, and lift your upper body and knees off the ground simultaneously. Focus on controlled movements and maintaining a diagonal V shape. Start with 3 sets of 5 reps per side.
- **Assisted V abs:** Use a stable object like a bench or wall to assist your initial lift, gradually reducing your reliance on it as you build strength. This helps focus on the core movement without overwhelming your muscles.

Step 3: Conquer the V abs Summit:

With a strong foundation and practiced components, you're ready to climb the V abs mountain! Start with:

- **Modified V abs:** Lie on your side, engage your core, and lift your upper body off the ground while keeping your legs straight but extended on the floor. Slowly lower back down with control. Do 3 sets of 5 reps per side.
- **Full V abs:** Gradually transition to full V abs, lifting both your upper body and legs off the ground simultaneously. Maintain a controlled movement, engage your core throughout, and prioritize form over speed. Start with 3 sets of 3-5 reps per side.

Remember:

- **Listen to your body:** Don't push yourself to pain or discomfort. If you feel any pain, stop and consult a healthcare professional.
- **Progress gradually:** Increase reps, sets, or difficulty as you get stronger. Don't rush the process.
- **Focus on form:** Proper technique is crucial to avoid injury and maximize benefits.

- **Celebrate your progress:** Every conquered rep is a step closer to your goal. Be proud of your hard work!

With dedication and these progressions, you'll be well on your way to mastering the V abs and unlocking a stronger, more sculpted core. Remember, the journey is just as important as the destination, so enjoy the climb!

Chapter 5

Variations of the Oblique V abs

Weighted Oblique V abs: Level Up Your Core Challenge (But Proceed with Caution!)

Mastered the basic V abs and craving a bigger core challenge? Weighted oblique V abs might seem like the next logical step, but before you reach for the dumbbells, **proceed with caution**. While adding weight can increase the intensity and effectiveness of the exercise, improper form or premature introduction can lead to injury.

Benefits of Weighted Oblique V abs:

- **Increased muscle engagement:** Adding weight challenges your core muscles further, leading to faster strength and definition gains.
- **Improved core stability:** The extra weight demands greater core stability to

maintain proper form, enhancing overall core function.

- **Boosted metabolic rate:** Lifting weights increases your overall energy expenditure, potentially supporting fat burning and weight management.

Risks and Considerations:

- **Increased injury risk:** Improper form with weights is far more dangerous than with bodyweight V abs. Ensure you have mastered the basic technique before adding weight.
- **Spine strain:** Improper weight distribution or excessive weight can put undue stress on your spine, leading to pain or injury.
- **Not suitable for everyone:** Individuals with pre-existing back problems, limited core strength, or mobility issues should avoid weighted V abs.

Safety First:

- **Master the basics:** Before adding weight, ensure you can perform bodyweight V abs with perfect form and controlled movements.
- **Start light:** Begin with the lightest possible weight (like a small water bottle) and gradually increase as your strength improves.
- **Focus on form:** Never sacrifice form for weight. It's better to use lighter weights with perfect technique than risk injury with heavier weights.
- **Listen to your body:** Stop immediately if you experience any pain or discomfort.
- **Seek professional guidance:** If you're unsure about weighted V abs, consult a certified trainer or physical therapist for personalized advice and instruction.

Alternative Progressions:

- **Increase reps and sets:** Instead of adding weight, consider increasing the number of reps and sets in your bodyweight V abs routine for a gradual challenge.

- **Try variations:** Explore more challenging V abs variations like Russian twists with a weight, medicine ball throws with a twist, or weighted side planks.
- **Focus on other core exercises:** Don't neglect other core exercises that can strengthen your core effectively without the increased risk of weighted V abs.

Remember: Building a strong, functional core takes time and dedication. Prioritize proper form, listen to your body, and explore alternative progressions before diving into weighted V abs. Your core will thank you for it!

Decline Oblique V abs: The Advanced Climber's Challenge

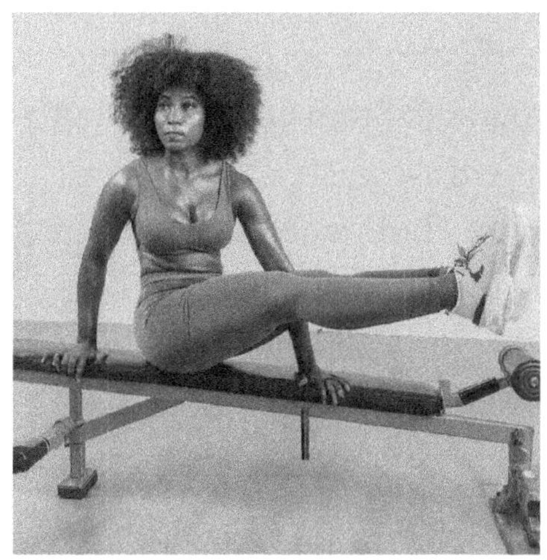

Conquered the basic V abs and its weighted variations? Ready to push your core to new heights? Enter the **decline oblique V abs**, a challenging exercise that takes core activation to the next level. But remember, this is for **advanced climbers only**, requiring proper technique and core strength to avoid injury.

Benefits of Decline Oblique V abs:

- **Increased core activation:** The decline position increases the leverage, forcing your core muscles to work harder, leading to faster strength and definition gains.

- **Enhanced rotational power:** This exercise specifically targets your obliques, crucial for rotational movements in sports and daily activities.
- **Advanced core challenge:** Decline V abs provide a significant challenge for seasoned exercisers, pushing your core strength and stability to the limit.

Considerations and Risks:

- **Highly advanced:** This exercise is not suitable for beginners or those with weak core muscles, due to the increased difficulty and injury risk.
- **Requires perfect form:** Improper technique can put undue stress on your spine and lead to pain or injury. Ensure you've mastered the basic V abs with flawless form before attempting the decline version.

- **Limited equipment needed:** While a decline bench is ideal, you can improvise with an inclined bench or sturdy incline.

Safe Execution:

- **Warm up thoroughly:** Prepare your core with dynamic stretches and light core exercises before tackling the decline V abs.
- **Start light:** If using weights, begin with very light weights like small dumbbells or medicine balls. Focus on form, not weight.
- **Control is key:** Perform the movement slowly and with control throughout the entire range of motion. Avoid jerky movements.
- **Engage your core:** Remember, this is all about core activation. Squeeze your obliques throughout the V abs and maintain a flat back.
- **Listen to your body:** Stop immediately if you experience any pain or discomfort. Don't push your limits.

Progression Tips:

- **Master bodyweight decline V abs:** Before adding weight, ensure you can perform decline V abs with perfect form using your bodyweight alone.
- **Increase difficulty gradually:** Once comfortable with bodyweight reps, consider adding light weights, starting with one weight in each hand.
- **Explore variations:** Try different arm positions, like holding the weight behind your head or overhead, to challenge your core in different ways.
- **Prioritize safety:** Always prioritize proper form over adding weight or difficulty. It's better to do fewer reps with perfect technique than risk injury.

Remember: Mastering the decline oblique V abs takes time, dedication, and a strong foundation. Don't rush the process, focus on safe execution, and enjoy the challenge! If you're unsure about this exercise, consult a certified trainer or physical therapist for personalized guidance.

This chapter concludes your journey through the world of V abs, from beginner progressions to advanced variations. Remember, a strong core is essential for overall health, fitness, and injury prevention. Choose the exercises that suit your current fitness level and goals, and most importantly, listen to your body and enjoy the process!

Hanging Oblique V abs: The Aerial Core Challenge (For the Fearless Climbers)

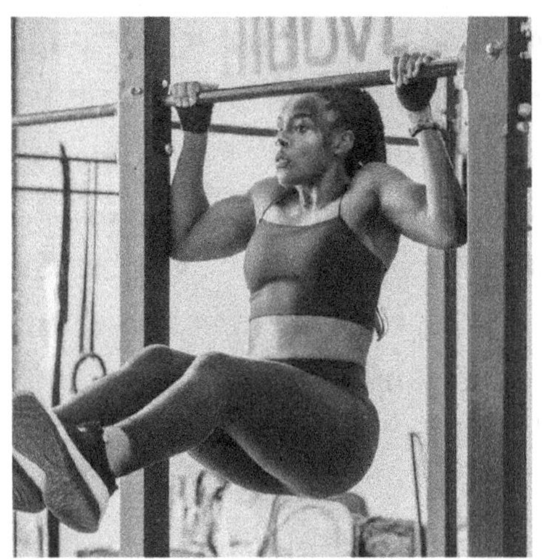

Ready to take your core strength and grip to new heights? Look no further than the **hanging oblique V abs**, the ultimate test of core control and upper body power. But be warned, this exercise demands advanced strength, perfect technique, and a healthy dose of courage – it's not for the faint of heart!

Benefits of Hanging Oblique V abs:

- **Ultimate core activation:** The hanging position intensifies the exercise, forcing your core muscles to work even harder, leading to significant strength and definition gains.

- **Enhanced functional core:** This exercise translates directly to improved core stability and power for various athletic activities and daily movements.
- **Grip strength boost:** Holding onto the bar challenges your grip strength, adding an extra layer of difficulty and benefit.
- **Advanced core challenge:** This exercise pushes your core and grip strength to the limit, providing a rewarding challenge for seasoned exercisers.

Considerations and Risks:

- **Extremely advanced:** This exercise requires exceptional core strength, grip strength, and coordination. It's not suitable for beginners or those with limited core strength or upper body power.
- **High injury risk:** Improper technique or attempting the exercise before you're

ready can lead to serious injuries like shoulder or spinal strain.

- **Requires specific equipment:** You'll need a pull-up bar with enough space to swing your legs without hitting anything.

Safe Execution:

- **Master basic V abs:** Before attempting hanging V abs, ensure you can perform regular V abs on the ground with perfect form and controlled movements.
- **Build grip strength:** Gradually strengthen your grip with exercises like pull-ups, dead hangs, or farmer's carries before attempting hanging V abs.
- **Warm up thoroughly:** Prepare your core and upper body with dynamic stretches and light exercises before tackling this challenging move.
- **Start with assisted reps:** Use resistance bands or a partner to assist you in the initial lift until you build enough strength to perform full reps independently.

- **Focus on form:** Maintain a flat back, engage your core throughout, and control the movement both upwards and downwards. Avoid swinging or jerking your body.
- **Know your limits:** Don't attempt this exercise if you're not confident in your core strength or grip. Listen to your body and stop immediately if you experience any pain or discomfort.

Progression Tips:

- **Master bodyweight hanging V abs:** Before adding weight, focus on perfecting the hanging V abs with your bodyweight only.
- **Gradually increase reps and sets:** Once comfortable with bodyweight reps, slowly increase the number of reps and sets you can perform with good form.
- **Explore weighted variations:** Once you've mastered bodyweight reps, consider adding light weights in your hands or ankles, starting with very light

weights and gradually increasing as your strength improves.

- **Focus on safety:** Always prioritize proper form and controlled movements over adding weight or difficulty. It's better to do fewer reps safely than risk injury.

Remember: Hanging oblique V abs are an advanced exercise with inherent risks. Consult a certified trainer or physical therapist for personalized guidance before attempting this move, especially if you have any pre-existing conditions or limitations.

This concludes your exploration of the V abs world, from beginner progressions to the ultimate hanging challenge. Remember, core strength is crucial for overall health and fitness. Choose exercises that suit your fitness level and goals, prioritize safety, and enjoy the journey towards a stronger, healthier you!

Beyond the Basics: Exploring Creative V abs Variations

The world of V abs goes beyond the standard exercises you've already explored. If you're looking for ways to keep your core challenged and engaged, dive into these creative variations:

Weighted variations:

- **Plate V abs:** Lie on a decline bench with a weight plate held behind your head. Perform V abs while keeping the plate close to your head throughout the movement. Start light and progress gradually.

- **Sandbag V abs:** Place a sandbag on your chest and perform V abs. The uneven weight distribution challenges your core stability and obliques in new ways.

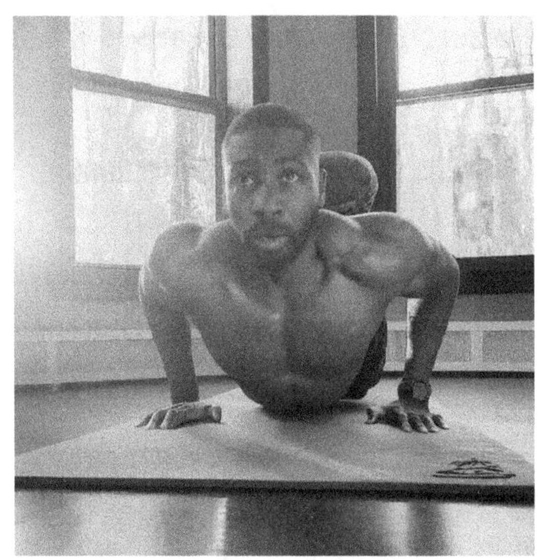

- **Single-leg V abs:** Hold a dumbbell in one hand and extend the opposite leg straight as you lift your torso off the ground. This variation intensifies core engagement and challenges your balance.

Explosive variations:

- **Tuck jumps with V abs:** Perform a jump squat, bringing your knees towards your chest, and explosively extend your legs and torso into a V abs at the peak of the jump. This adds a plyometric element to your core workout.

- **Box jumps with V abs:** Jump onto a sturdy box and immediately transition into a V abs at the top. This exercise requires power and core control for landing safely.
- **Jump rope V abs:** Alternate jump rope jumps with V abs, maintaining a continuous rhythm. This keeps your heart rate up while challenging your core coordination.

Stability variations:

- **Swiss ball V abs:** Lie on a Swiss ball with your lower back and legs supported. Perform V abs while maintaining core engagement and stability on the ball. This challenges your core and balance simultaneously.
- **Bosu ball V abs:** Place your feet on a Bosu ball (dome side down) and perform V abs. The unstable surface requires constant core activation to maintain balance.

- **Anti-rotational V abs:** Lie on your side with a medicine ball held at your chest. As you lift your torso, resist the urge to rotate your hips; focus on keeping your core engaged and body stable.

Remember:

- **Choose variations that suit your fitness level and limitations.**
- **Prioritize proper form over speed or difficulty.**
- **Start light and gradually increase intensity as you get stronger.**
- **Listen to your body and stop if you experience any pain or discomfort.**
- **Consult a certified trainer or physical therapist if you have any concerns or pre-existing conditions.**

With these creative variations and safety guidelines in mind, you can keep your V abs routine fresh, challenging, and effective, unlocking a stronger and more sculpted core along the way!

Chapter 6

Designing an Oblique V abs Training Program

Setting goals and defining success are crucial steps in any fitness journey, including mastering V abs. Here's a framework to help you create a personalized plan:

1. Identify Your "Why":

- What motivates you to improve your core strength and V abs skills? Do you want a more defined core, better athletic performance, or improved everyday movement? Identifying your "why" keeps you focused and motivated during challenging workouts.

2. Set SMART Goals:

- **Specific:** Clearly define what you want to achieve, e.g., "Perform 10 full V abs with perfect form in 3 months."

- **Measurable:** Choose quantifiable metrics to track your progress, e.g., number of reps, sets, or completion time.
- **Achievable:** Set realistic goals based on your current fitness level and gradually increase difficulty as you improve.
- **Relevant:** Ensure your goals align with your overall fitness goals and "why."
- **Time-bound:** Set a timeframe for achieving your goals to stay accountable.

3. Define Success in Your Terms:

- Success isn't just about reaching the final goal. Celebrate smaller milestones along the way, like mastering a new variation or increasing your rep count.
- Focus on progress, not perfection. Everyone has setbacks, but celebrating effort and consistency is key.
- Define success beyond physical achievements. Maybe it's increased confidence, improved posture, or feeling more empowered in your body.

4. Create an Action Plan:

- Break down your main goal into smaller, actionable steps. For example, if your goal is 10 V abs, start with bodyweight progressions, gradually add weight, and practice specific variations.
- Schedule your workouts and stick to a consistent routine, allowing for rest and recovery days.
- Find a workout buddy or accountability partner to support and motivate you.

5. Track Your Progress:

- Keep a workout journal or use a fitness app to track your reps, sets, and any personal notes about your workouts.
- Regularly review your progress to identify areas for improvement and celebrate your achievements.
- Remember, progress isn't always linear. Don't get discouraged by plateaus; focus on maintaining effort and consistency.

6. Enjoy the Journey:

- Exercise should be enjoyable! Find V abs variations you like, incorporate fun music, and focus on moving your body with intention and joy.
- Celebrate the positive changes you experience, both physical and mental.
- Embrace the challenge and remember that even small steps lead to big results!

By setting clear goals, defining success in your terms, and creating an actionable plan, you can conquer your V abs journey and achieve a stronger, healthier core. Remember, consistency and self-compassion are key ingredients to reaching your fitness goals and enjoying the process along the way!

Choosing the right reps, sets, and tempo for your V abs routine depends on your individual goals and fitness level. Here's a guide to help you personalize your workout:

Based on your goals:

- **Strength and muscle definition:** Aim for **lower reps (8-12) with heavier weights (optional) and slower tempos (3-4 seconds up, 3-4 seconds down).** Rest for 30-60 seconds between sets.
- **Endurance and core stability:** Opt for **higher reps (15-20) with lighter weights or bodyweight only and moderate tempos (2-3 seconds up, 2-3 seconds down).** Rest for 15-30 seconds between sets.
- **Beginner focus:** Start with **bodyweight V abs, focusing on mastering proper form with controlled movements.** Aim for 3-5 reps per set and gradually increase as you get stronger. Rest for 30-60 seconds between sets.

Based on your fitness level:

- **Beginner:** 2-3 sets of 5-10 reps, slower tempos, lighter weights (optional).
- **Intermediate:** 3-4 sets of 10-15 reps, moderate tempos, moderate weights (optional).
- **Advanced:** 4-5 sets of 15-20 reps, faster tempos, heavier weights (optional).

Remember:

- **Listen to your body:** Adjust reps, sets, and tempo based on how you feel. Don't push yourself to pain or discomfort.
- **Focus on form over speed:** It's better to perform fewer reps with perfect form than many reps with compromised technique.
- **Warm up and cool down:** Prepare your body with dynamic stretches before and static stretches after your workout.
- **Progress gradually:** Don't increase intensity or difficulty too quickly to avoid injury.

- **Consult a professional:** If you have any concerns or pre-existing conditions, consult a certified trainer or physical therapist for personalized guidance.

Additional tips:

- **Incorporate different variations:** Add variety to your workout with different V abs variations like weighted, decline, or medicine ball versions.
- **Supersets or circuits:** Combine V abs with other core exercises like planks, side planks, or Russian twists for a more efficient workout.
- **Track your progress:** Monitor your reps, sets, and workout times to see your improvement and adjust your routine as needed.

Remember, there's no one-size-fits-all answer. Experiment with different combinations of reps, sets, and tempos to find what works best for you and helps you achieve your V abs goals safely and effectively!

Integrating V abs into your workout routine effectively depends on your individual fitness level, goals, and overall training plan. Here's a guide to help you find the right frequency and integration strategy:

Frequency:

- **Beginner:** Start with 2-3 V abs sessions per week, allowing at least 1-2 rest days between sessions for muscle recovery. Focus on mastering proper form before increasing frequency.
- **Intermediate:** Aim for 3-4 sessions per week, with rest days strategically placed depending on the intensity of your other workouts.
- **Advanced:** You can potentially train V abs daily, but ensure adequate rest and recovery, consider incorporating active recovery sessions, and listen closely to your body for any signs of overuse.

Integration:

- **Warm-up:** Light V abs with bodyweight can be a great way to activate your core before your main workout, especially if it involves core-intensive exercises.
- **Standalone core workout:** Dedicate a specific workout session to core exercises, including various V abs variations, planks, and other core-strengthening moves.
- **Circuit training:** Combine V abs with other exercises like squats, lunges, or push-ups for a full-body circuit workout that challenges both strength and endurance.
- **HIIT workouts:** Include explosive V abs variations like jump rope V abs or box jumps with V abs for a high-intensity interval training session that boosts core power and cardio fitness.

Important factors to consider:

- **Overall training volume:** If you already engage in other demanding workouts, adjust your V abs frequency to avoid overtraining your core.

- **Recovery:** Prioritize rest and recovery days to allow your muscles to rebuild and prevent injuries.
- **Listen to your body:** Pain, soreness, or fatigue are signs you might need to adjust your frequency or intensity.
- **Seek professional guidance:** If you're unsure about proper integration, consult a certified trainer or physical therapist for personalized advice.

Remember: Consistency is key. Regularly incorporating V abs into your routine, even if it's just a few reps a day, will lead to long-term core strength and stability improvements. Enjoy the process, experiment with different approaches, and listen to your body for optimal results!

Sample V abs Training Programs for Different Fitness Levels:

Beginner:

- **Frequency:** 2-3 times per week
- **Warm-up:** 5-10 minutes of light cardio and dynamic stretches
- **Workout:**
  - **Bodyweight V abs:** 3 sets of 5-8 reps, rest 30-60 seconds between sets
  - **Plank:** 3 sets of 30-second holds, rest 30 seconds between sets
  - **Bird-dog:** 3 sets of 10 reps per side, rest 30 seconds between sets
- **Cool-down:** 5-10 minutes of static stretches

Intermediate:

- **Frequency:** 3-4 times per week
- **Warm-up:** 5-10 minutes of light cardio and dynamic stretches
- **Workout:**

- o **Knee-up V abs:** 3 sets of 10-12 reps, rest 30 seconds between sets
  - o **Side plank with hip dips:** 3 sets of 10-12 reps per side, rest 30 seconds between sets
  - o **Weighted Russian twists:** 3 sets of 10-15 reps per side, rest 30 seconds between sets (start with light weight)
- **Cool-down:** 5-10 minutes of static stretches

Advanced:

- **Frequency:** 4-5 times per week
- **Warm-up:** 5-10 minutes of light cardio and dynamic stretches
- **Workout:**
  - o **Medicine ball oblique V abs:** 3 sets of 8-10 reps per side, rest 30 seconds between sets
  - o **Decline V abs:** 3 sets of 5-8 reps, rest 45-60 seconds between sets (use caution and proper form)

- ○ **Hanging leg raises:** 3 sets of 10-12 reps, rest 30 seconds between sets
- **Cool-down:** 5-10 minutes of static stretches

Remember:

- These are just samples; you can adjust the exercises, sets, reps, and rest times based on your individual needs and fitness level.
- Always prioritize proper form over speed or weight.
- Listen to your body and take rest days when needed.
- Consider consulting a certified trainer or physical therapist for personalized guidance, especially if you have any pre-existing conditions.

Additional Tips:

- You can add variety to your workouts by trying different V abs variations, using different equipment, or combining V abs with other core exercises.

- Track your progress so you can see how you're improving over time.
- Most importantly, have fun and enjoy the challenge!

V abs Workout Log Sheet

This log sheet can help you track your progress and stay motivated as you work towards your V abs goals. Feel free to customize it to fit your needs.

Date:

Goal: (e.g., number of reps, specific variation)

Warm-up: (brief description of warm-up exercises)

Workout:

Cool-down: (brief description of cool-down exercises)

Overall feeling: (e.g., easy, challenging, sore)

Additional notes:

Tips:

- Use different colors or symbols to highlight different types of exercises.

- Track your progress over time to see how you're improving.
- Use the notes section to record any specific observations or challenges you experience.
- Share your log sheet with a friend or trainer for accountability and support.

https://docs.google.com/spreadsheets/d/1NLZwFkqhy5dCgC9QmbgkNv3Ps1SdAMtVLZc-krqM0Yc/edit?usp=drivesdk
Link for sample Workout log sheet

Chapter 7

Supersets, drop sets, and other advanced training methods

Supersets, drop sets, and other advanced training methods can be effective tools for experienced lifters seeking to break plateaus, boost intensity, and improve muscle endurance. However, they're not without their drawbacks and should be used strategically for optimal results. Here's a breakdown of each method:

Supersets:

- **What they are:** Combining two exercises back-to-back with minimal rest (10-30 seconds). Typically, exercises target opposing muscle groups (e.g., chest press + rows), but agonist-antagonist pairings (e.g., bicep curls + tricep extensions) are also used.

- **Benefits:** Increased intensity, time efficiency, improved cardiovascular fitness, potential for greater calorie burn.
- **Drawbacks:** Requires good form and control, can be fatiguing, not ideal for building pure strength.

Drop sets:

- **What they are:** Reducing the weight used throughout a set while maintaining the reps and decreasing rest (minimal or none). Can be achieved by pre-loading weights on the bar or having lighter dumbbells ready.
- **Benefits:** Increases muscle fatigue, targets additional muscle fibers, can help overcome sticking points.
- **Drawbacks:** Can compromise form if not done carefully, not ideal for beginners, potential for overtraining.

Other advanced methods:

- **Giant sets:** Similar to supersets, but involving 3 or more exercises back-to-back. Offers even higher intensity but comes with increased fatigue and form risk.
- **Pre-exhaust and post-exhaust:** Pre-exhausting a muscle group with an isolation exercise before a compound movement, or vice versa. Can prioritize specific muscle groups but adds complexity and time.
- **Negatives:** Focusing on the lowering portion of a lift with heavier weights than you can lift concentrically. Highly stressful on muscles and joints, use cautiously.

Remember:

- These methods are for experienced lifters with good form and understanding of their bodies.
- Consult a certified trainer for personalized guidance and ensure proper technique to avoid injury.

- Don't rely solely on advanced methods; incorporate them strategically within a balanced training program.
- Prioritize proper form over heavier weights or faster tempos.
- Listen to your body and take rest days when needed.

Additional tips:

- Start with lighter weights and lower reps when trying new methods.
- Experiment with different variations and find what works best for you.
- Track your progress and adjust your routine based on your goals and responses.

Overall, supersets, drop sets, and other advanced techniques can be valuable tools for experienced lifters, but use them carefully and strategically within a well-structured training program for optimal results and injury prevention.

Periodization is a crucial approach for any lifter or exerciser seeking long-term progress. It involves strategically planning your workouts in phases with varying intensity, volume, and focus to optimize adaptation and prevent plateaus. Here's a breakdown of periodization for V abs training:

Phases:

1. Preparatory Phase (2-4 weeks):

- **Goal:** Build a strong foundation and prepare your body for more demanding work.
- **Focus:** Moderate intensity, higher reps (12-15), lower weights (bodyweight or light), more frequent sessions (3-4 times per week).
- **Example:** Bodyweight V abs, plank variations, bird-dogs, light medicine ball throws with V abs.

2. Strength Phase (4-6 weeks):

- **Goal:** Increase maximal strength and muscle mass in your core.
- **Focus:** Higher intensity, lower reps (8-12), heavier weights (gradually increase), moderate frequency (3-4 times per week).
- **Example:** Weighted V abs (start light), decline V abs (advanced), hanging leg raises, weighted Russian twists.

3. Hypertrophy Phase (4-6 weeks):

- **Goal:** Increase core muscle size and definition.
- **Focus:** Moderate intensity, moderate-high reps (10-15), moderate weights (challenging but controllable), higher frequency (4-5 times per week).
- **Example:** Supersets of V abs variations, drop sets on decline V abs, AMRAP (as many reps as possible) sets with bodyweight V abs, cable crunches.

4. Transition Phase (2-3 weeks):

- **Goal:** Gradually reduce training volume
  and intensity to allow for recovery and
  prepare for the next cycle.
- **Focus:** Lower intensity, moderate reps
  (10-12), lighter weights, lower frequency
  (2-3 times per week).
- **Example:** Bodyweight V abs, plank
  variations, light core circuits, active
  recovery exercises.

Remember:

- Periodization is a flexible framework;
  adjust duration and specific exercises
  based on your goals and experience.
- Deload weeks (taking a complete break or
  significantly reducing training) can be
  incorporated between phases for optimal
  recovery.
- Track your progress (reps, sets, weights)
  to monitor improvement and adjust the
  plan as needed.
- Consider consulting a certified trainer or
  physical therapist for a personalized
  periodization program.

Additional tips:

- Incorporate proper warm-up and cool-down before and after each training session.
- Prioritize proper form over heavier weights or faster tempos.
- Listen to your body and take rest days when needed.
- Stay motivated and enjoy the process of challenging yourself and seeing your core strength improve!

By implementing periodization principles into your V abs training, you can set yourself up for long-term progress, prevent plateaus, and achieve your core strength goals safely and effectively.

Common Pain Points in V abs Training and Solutions:

V abs can be a valuable exercise for core strength and stability, but they can also lead to pain if not performed correctly. Here are some common pain points and how to address them:

1. Lower Back Pain:

- **Cause:** Improper form, arching your back excessively, engaging your hip flexors instead of your core.
- **Solution:** Focus on keeping a flat back throughout the movement, engage your core by drawing your belly button towards your spine, don't lift your legs higher than your torso. Consider starting with easier progressions like planks or bird-dogs until you master the core engagement.

2. Neck Pain:

- **Cause:** Straining your neck by looking up or down excessively.

- **Solution:** Keep your neck in line with
  your spine throughout the movement, gaze
  slightly forward or keep your eyes focused
  on a fixed point in front of you.

3. Shoulder Pain:

- **Cause:** Swinging your momentum instead
  of using controlled movements, using
  weights that are too heavy.
- **Solution:** Avoid momentum, focus on
  slow and controlled movements, start with
  bodyweight and gradually increase weight
  as you get stronger, ensure proper
  shoulder alignment and don't round your
  shoulders.

4. Hip Pain:

- **Cause:** Overusing your hip flexors or
  straining your hip muscles due to
  improper form.
- **Solution:** Focus on engaging your core,
  not pulling your legs with your hip

flexors. Keep your legs straight and avoid excessive hip rotation.

5. Wrist Pain:

- **Cause:** Putting too much pressure on your wrists during planks or other supporting exercises.
- **Solution:** Ensure proper wrist alignment, distribute your weight evenly across your forearms, use padding if needed, consider modifying exercises if pain persists.

General Tips:

- **Warm up properly:** Include dynamic stretches and light cardio before your workout.
- **Listen to your body:** Don't push through pain, stop if you experience discomfort and adjust your technique or take a break.
- **Start with bodyweight:** Master the basic V abs with proper form before adding weight or variations.

- **Seek professional guidance:** If pain persists, consult a certified trainer or physical therapist for personalized advice and exercise modifications.

Remember, proper form is crucial for preventing pain and maximizing the benefits of V abs. Don't hesitate to adjust the exercises, modify the intensity, or seek professional help if needed to ensure a safe and effective workout experience.

Proper form:

- **Maximizes results:** Using the correct muscles and movement patterns ensures you target the intended areas and get the most out of your effort.
- **Reduces risk of injury:** Improper form can put unnecessary stress on joints, ligaments, and muscles, leading to pain and potential injuries.
- **Improves efficiency:** When you move correctly, you use your energy more effectively and can perform exercises for longer or with more weight.
- **Boosts confidence:** Knowing you're doing an exercise correctly can give you the confidence to push yourself further and enjoy your workout more.

Warm-up:

- **Prepares your body:** Gradually increases heart rate, blood flow, and muscle temperature, preventing injuries from sudden exertion.

- **Improves flexibility and range of motion:** Loosens up your muscles and joints, allowing for smoother and more efficient movement.
- **Activates the nervous system:** Alerts your body to prepare for physical activity, leading to better coordination and performance.
- **Reduces muscle soreness:** Proper warm-up can help minimize post-workout stiffness and discomfort.

Cool-down:

- **Gradually brings your body back to rest:** Allows your heart rate and blood pressure to decrease safely, preventing dizziness or lightheadedness.
- **Improves circulation and removes waste products:** Helps flush out lactic acid and other byproducts of exercise, potentially reducing muscle soreness.
- **Promotes flexibility and recovery:** Gentle stretches can help maintain

flexibility and prepare your body for
recovery.

- **Reduces risk of delayed onset muscle soreness (DOMS):** Proper cool-down can help minimize muscle soreness in the days following your workout.

Remember:

- **Every movement has proper form:** Whether it's V abs or any other exercise, take the time to learn and practice the correct technique.
- **Warm-up and cool-down are essential for every workout:** Don't skip them, even if you're short on time.
- **Listen to your body:** Adjust your exercise routine and intensity based on your individual needs and limitations.

By prioritizing proper form and incorporating thorough warm-up and cool-down routines, you can set yourself up for safe, effective, and enjoyable workouts that help you achieve your fitness goals.

Recognizing when to rest and when to seek professional guidance is crucial for any exerciser, especially when venturing into challenging exercises like V abs. Here's a framework to help you navigate these decisions:

Resting:

- **General fatigue:** Feeling tired or lacking motivation for several days in a row. Listen to your body and take a break to recharge.
- **Muscle soreness:** Mild soreness after a new or intense workout is normal. However, excessive or persistent soreness (DOMS) lasting several days could indicate overtraining. Rest and allow your muscles to recover.
- **Pain:** Acute pain during or after an exercise is a red flag. Stop immediately and rest the affected area. Seek professional advice if pain persists.
- **Plateauing progress:** Not seeing improvements despite consistent effort for weeks could indicate overtraining or

incorrect form. Consider rest, reassess your technique, or seek professional guidance.

- **Mental burnout:** Feeling stressed, anxious, or unmotivated towards exercise consistently. Prioritize mental well-being, take breaks, and consider activities you enjoy outside of structured workouts.

Seeking professional guidance:

- **Chronic pain:** If pain persists even after rest or modifies exercises, consult a doctor or physical therapist to rule out any underlying conditions and get personalized advice.
- **Pre-existing injuries or conditions:** If you have any concerns about how V abs or other exercises might affect your specific situation, a professional can guide you towards safe and effective exercise choices.
- **Difficulties mastering proper form:** If you struggle with proper form despite watching tutorials or reading instructions,

a trainer or physical therapist can provide
in-person feedback and adjustments.

- **Designing a personalized training
  program:** If you have specific goals and
  want a plan tailored to your needs and
  limitations, a professional can create a
  safe and effective program for you.
- **Motivation and accountability:** If you
  struggle with staying motivated or
  disciplined, a trainer can provide
  guidance, support, and accountability to
  help you reach your goals.

Remember:

- Taking rest days is crucial for recovery
  and preventing injuries.
- Pain is a signal to listen to your body and
  adjust your routine.
- Professional guidance can be invaluable
  for optimizing your workouts, addressing
  limitations, and reaching your fitness
  goals safely and effectively.

Don't hesitate to prioritize rest and seek professional help when needed. By respecting your body's limits and investing in your well-being, you can create a sustainable and enjoyable fitness journey that supports your long-term health and goals.

Bonus Materials

Appendix A: Anatomy charts and illustrations

here are some anatomy charts and illustrations of the muscles involved in V abs:

- **Anterior view of the trunk muscles:** This chart shows the rectus abdominis, the external obliques, and the internal obliques, which are all major muscles involved in V abs.

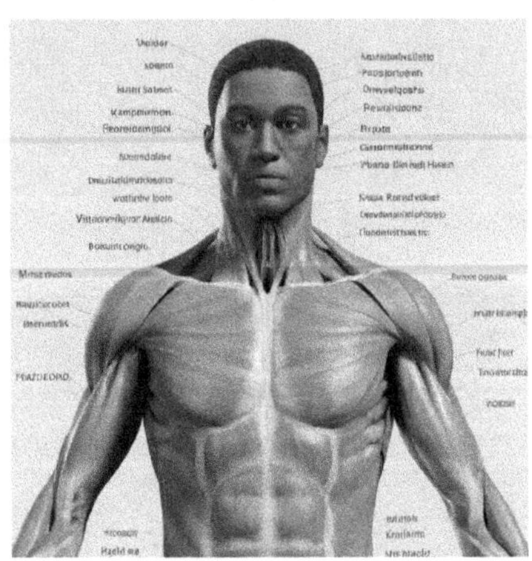

- **Posterior view of the trunk muscles:**
  This chart shows the erector spinae, which
  helps to support the spine during V abs.

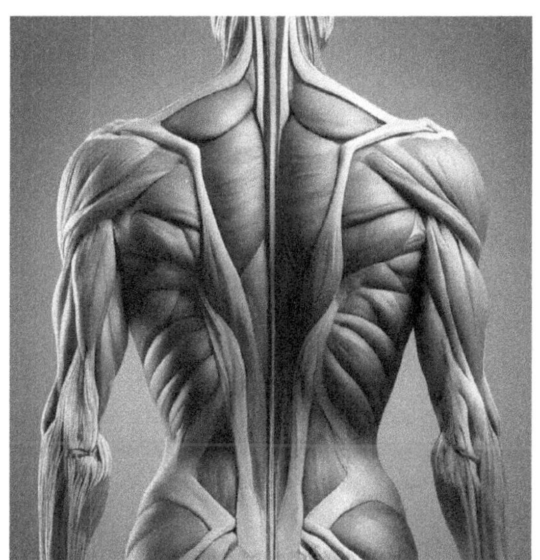

- **Lateral view of the trunk muscles:** This
  chart shows the obliques, which help to
  rotate the trunk during V abs

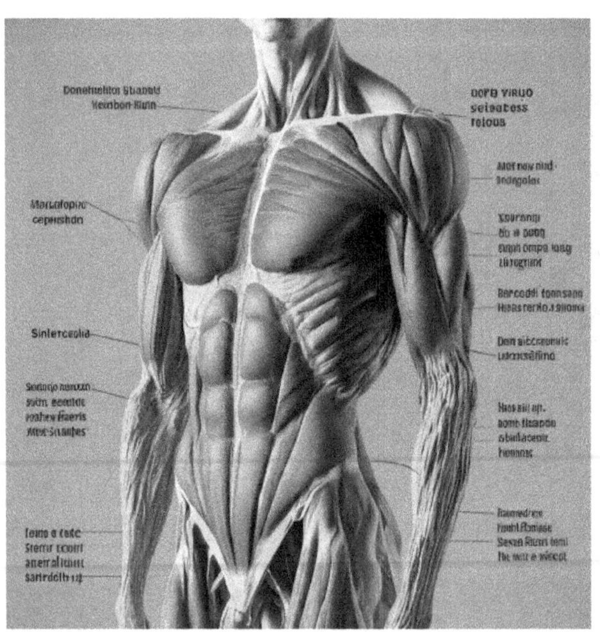

Diagram of the hip flexors: This diagram shows the iliopsoas, which is the main hip flexor muscle and helps to lift the legs during V abs.

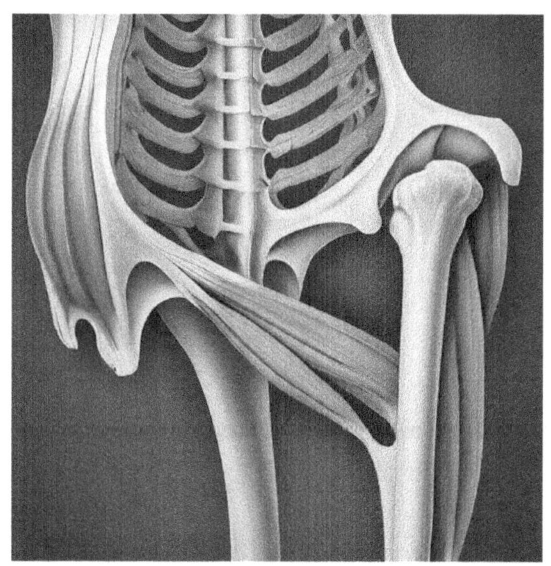

video demonstrations of various V abs variations:

https://screenpal.com/watch/cZnjqqVdOCH

Link for video tutorial

Conclusion

Mastering the V abs for a Strong Core

Your journey to mastering the V abs and achieving a strong core has been insightful! We've covered numerous aspects, from understanding the anatomy and muscle engagement to crafting a personalized training plan with progressions, variations, and periodization. Remember, the key takeaways are:

Prioritize proper form: Focus on controlled movements, engaging the correct muscles, and listening to your body to avoid injury. **Start with the basics:** Master the bodyweight V abs before adding weight or variations. **Progress gradually:** Increase difficulty slowly, allowing your body to adapt and prevent plateaus. **Warm up and cool down:** Prepare your muscles and prevent soreness with proper warm-up and cool-down routines. **Listen to your body:** Rest when needed, and seek professional guidance if you experience pain or have pre-existing conditions. **Enjoy the process:** Make your workouts fun and challenging, celebrate your progress, and track your achievements to stay motivated.

By staying informed, focusing on proper form, and implementing a tailored training plan, you can conquer the V abs and develop a strong, functional core that benefits your overall fitness and well-being. Remember, consistency and dedication are key, and I'm here to support you along the way!

Requesting a Review

I hope you're enjoying your journey towards oblique V abs mastery with my book "The Complete Guide to Oblique V abs: Mastering Technique, Variations, and Programming"!

I'm reaching out because your feedback is incredibly valuable to me as an author. It helps me understand what's working well in the guide and what areas I can improve for future editions.

If you've had a chance to read through the guide, I would be truly grateful if you could take a few minutes to leave a review . Even a short review sharing your thoughts on the clarity, helpfulness, and overall experience would be immensely helpful.

Here are some specific questions you might consider addressing in your review:

- Did you find the book easy to understand and follow?
- Were the explanations and instructions clear and concise?

- Did you find the different variations helpful and challenging?
- Did the book meet your expectations?
- Would you recommend this book to others?

Of course, any additional feedback you'd like to share is warmly welcome!

Thank you for your time and consideration. Your honest feedback is crucial in helping me grow as an author and provide even better resources for the fitness community.

Warmly,

Helen Talbott

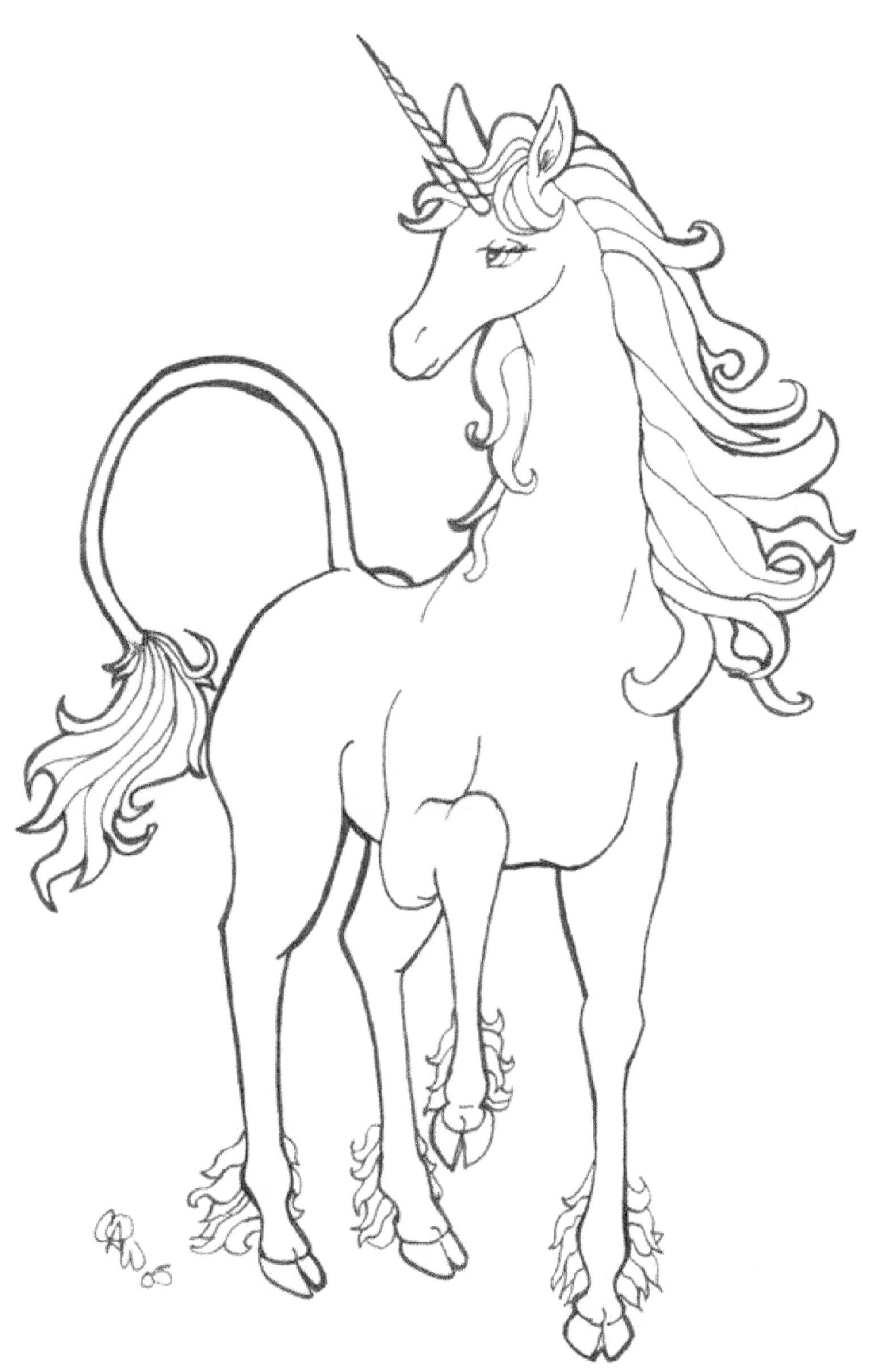

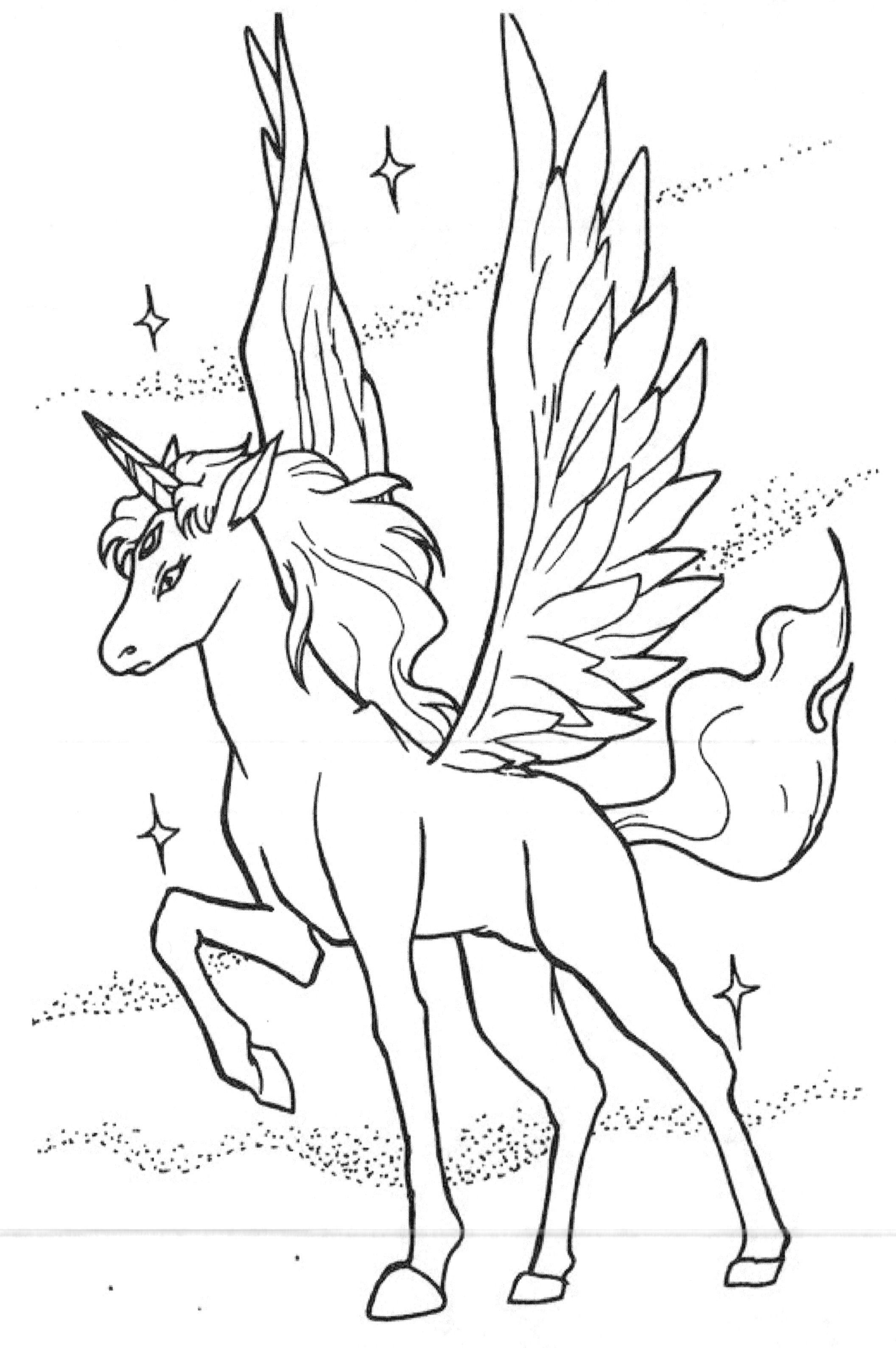

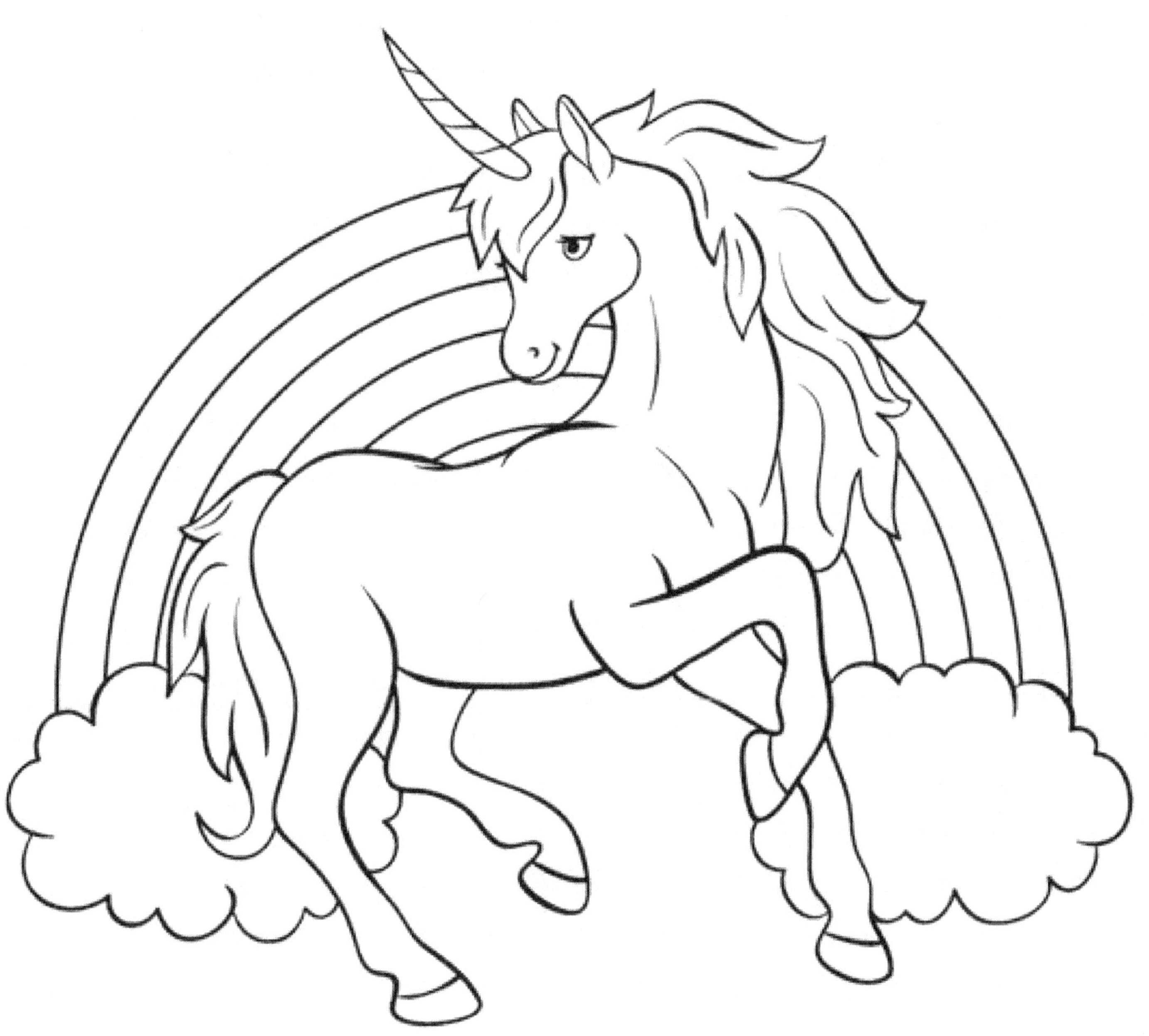

ColoringPages.Site

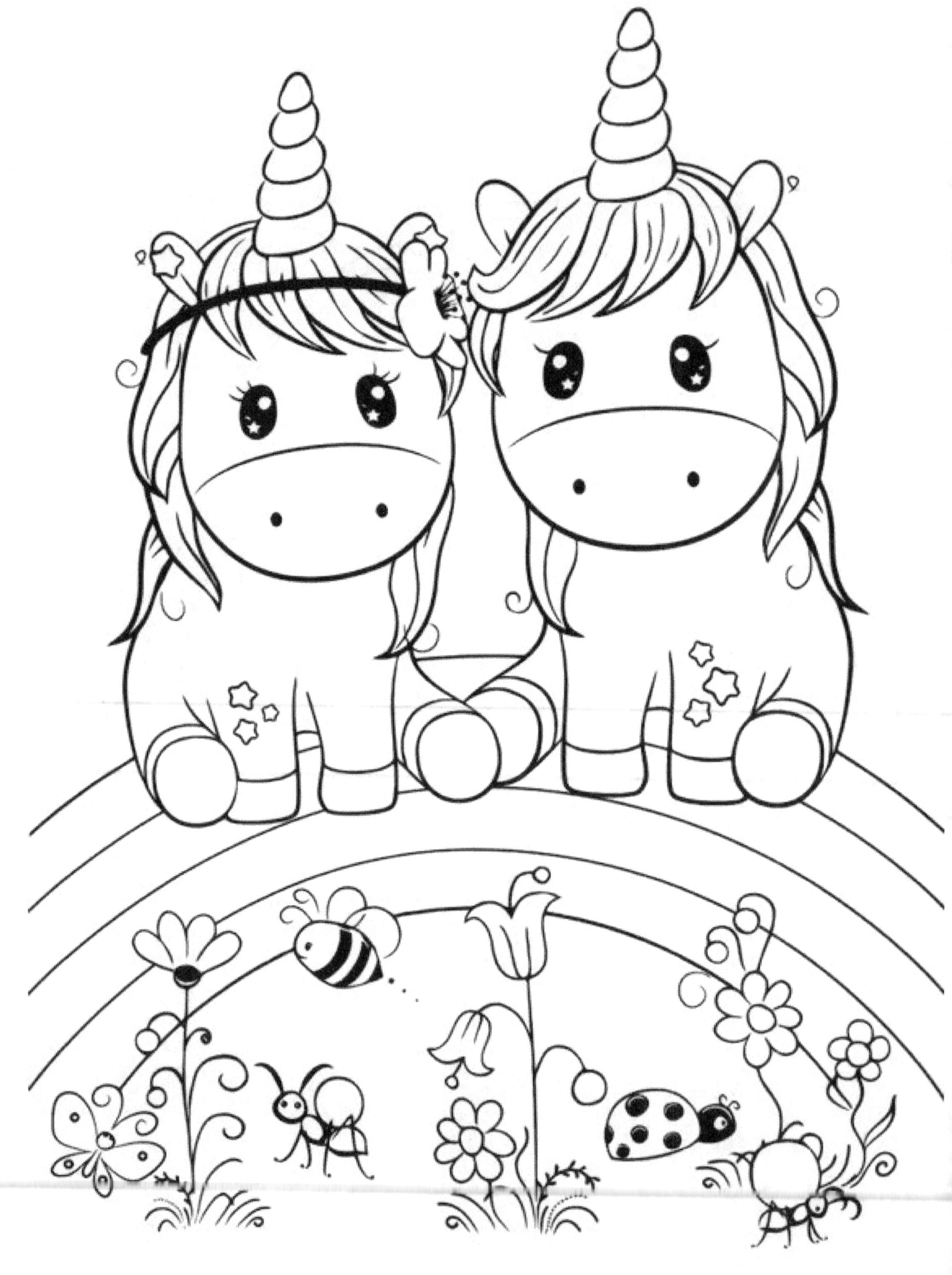

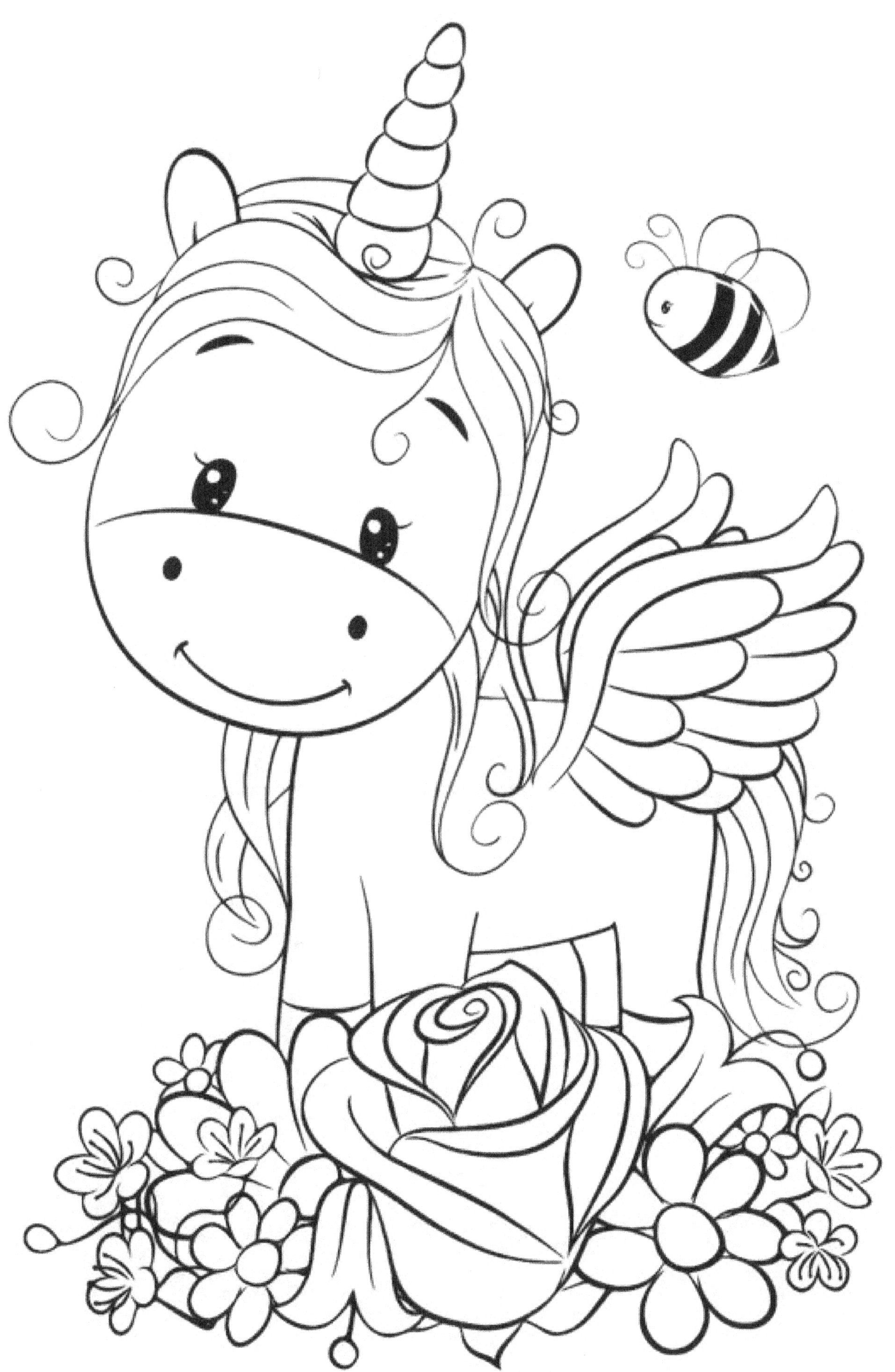

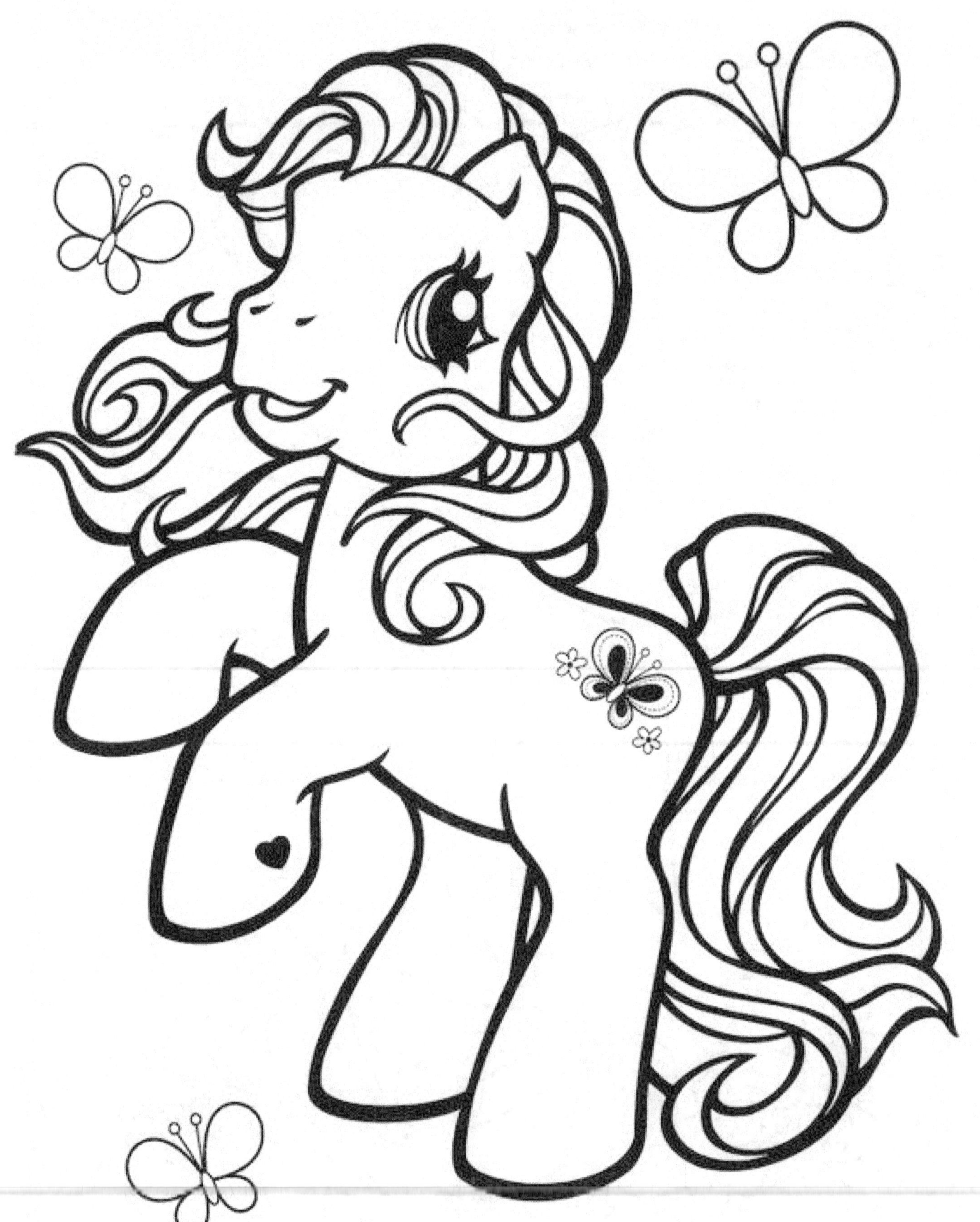

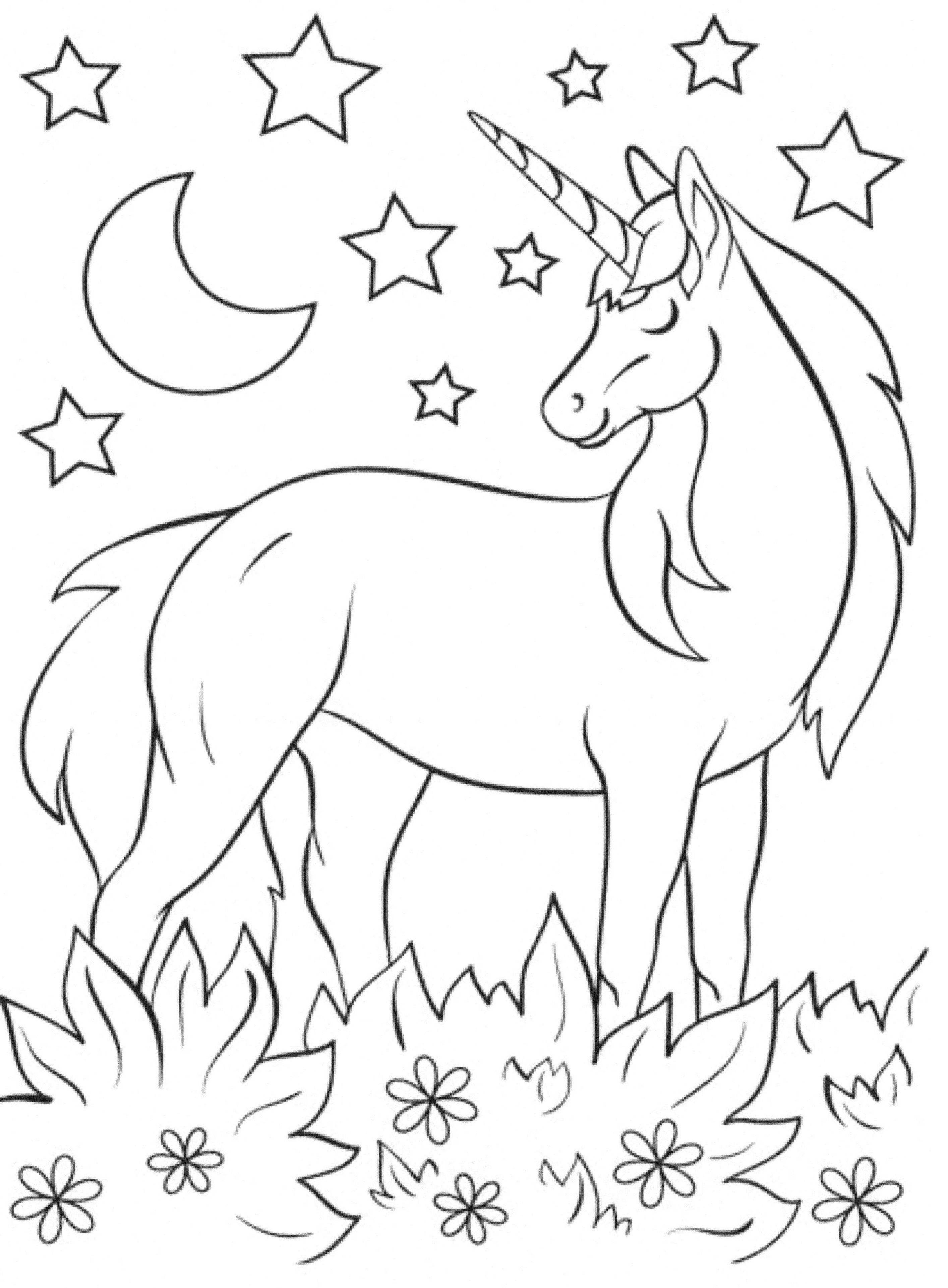

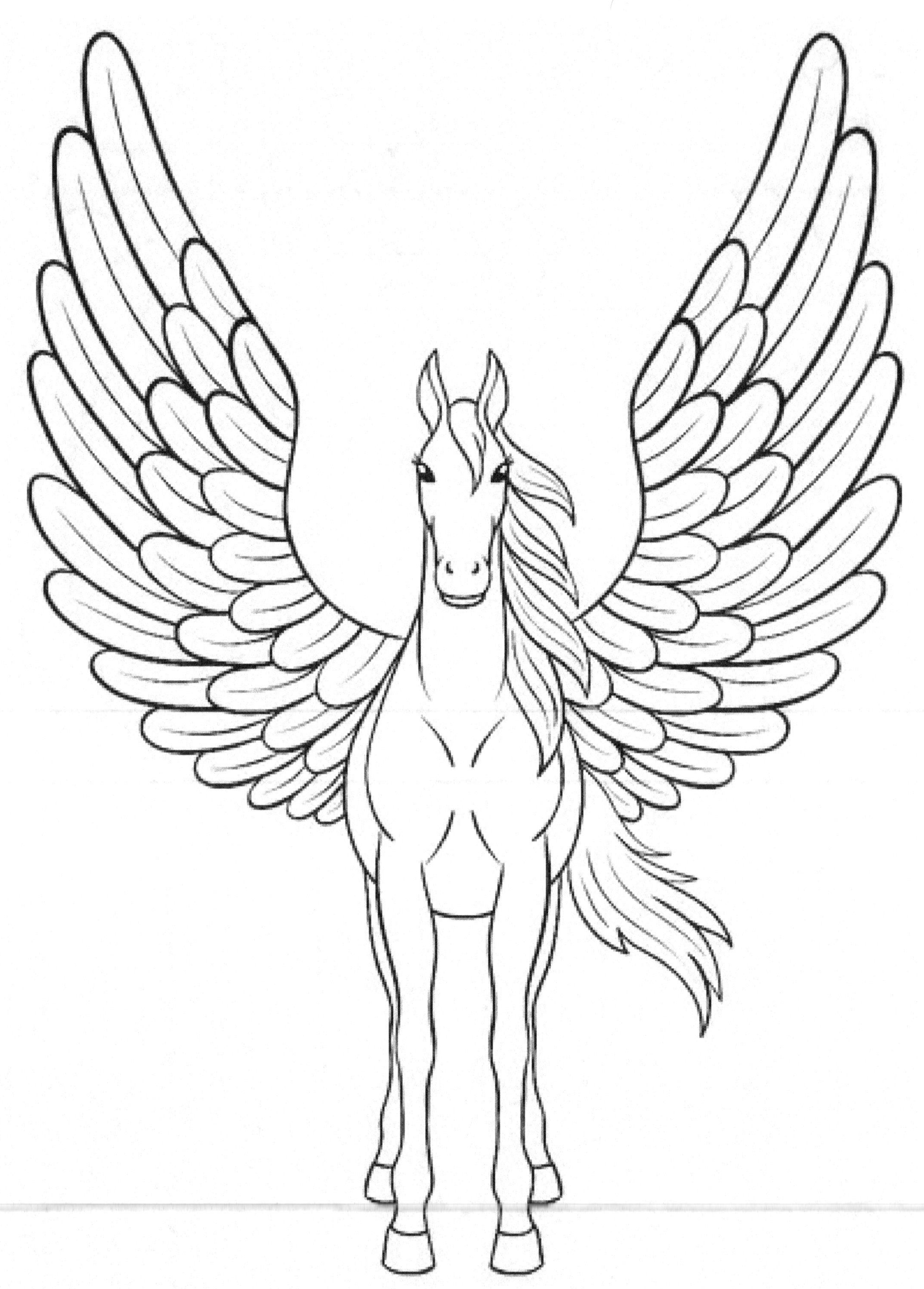

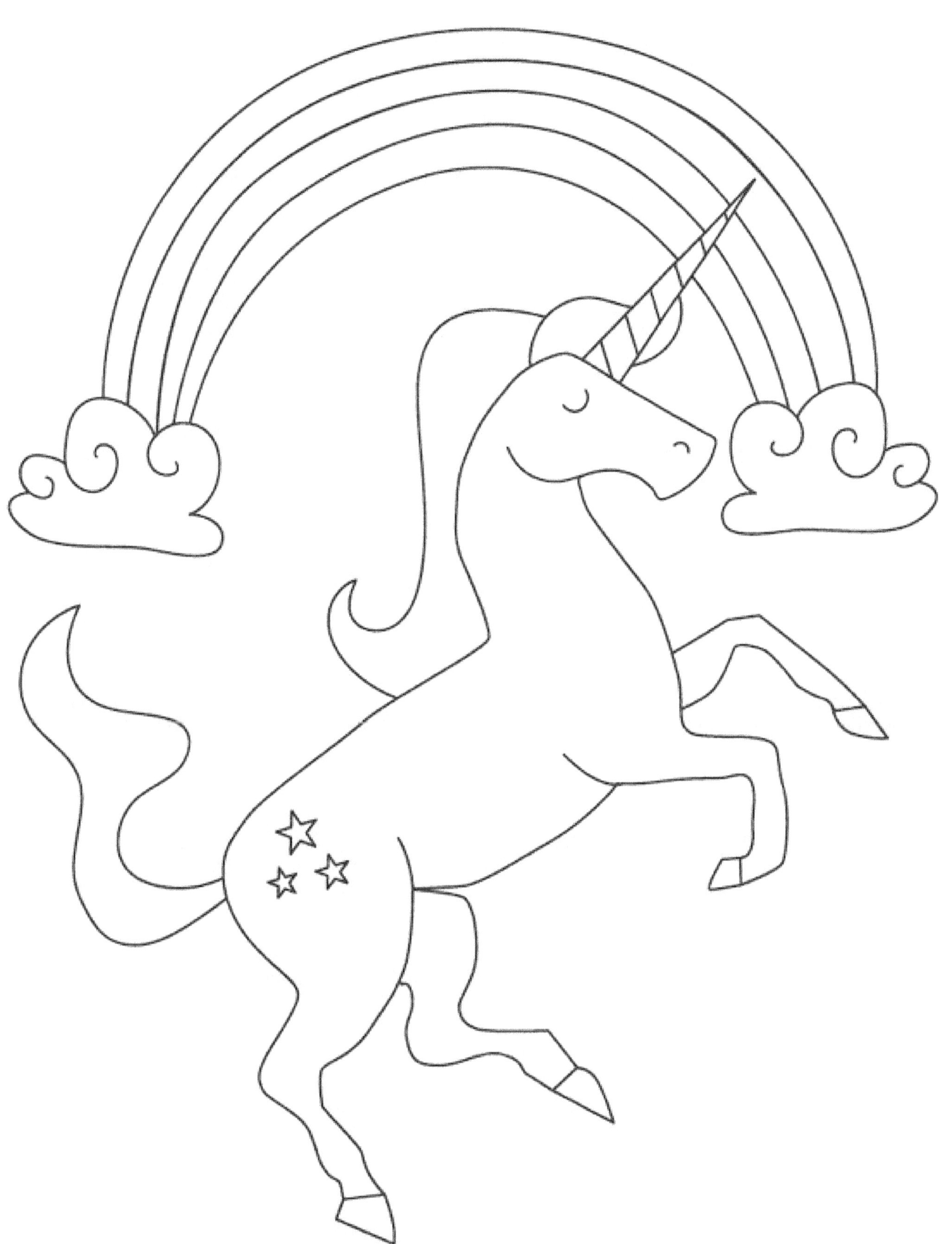

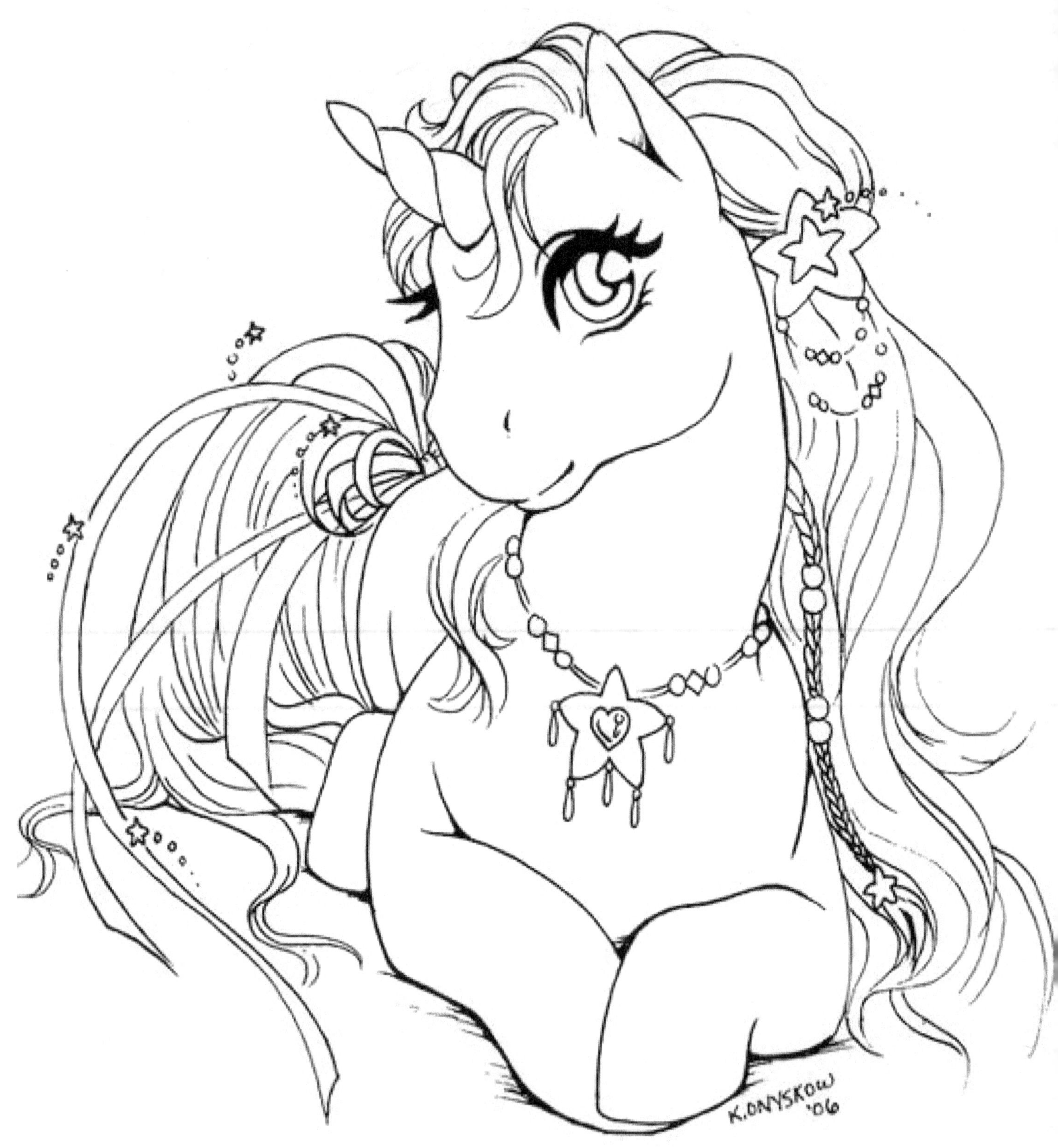
K.ONYSKOW '06

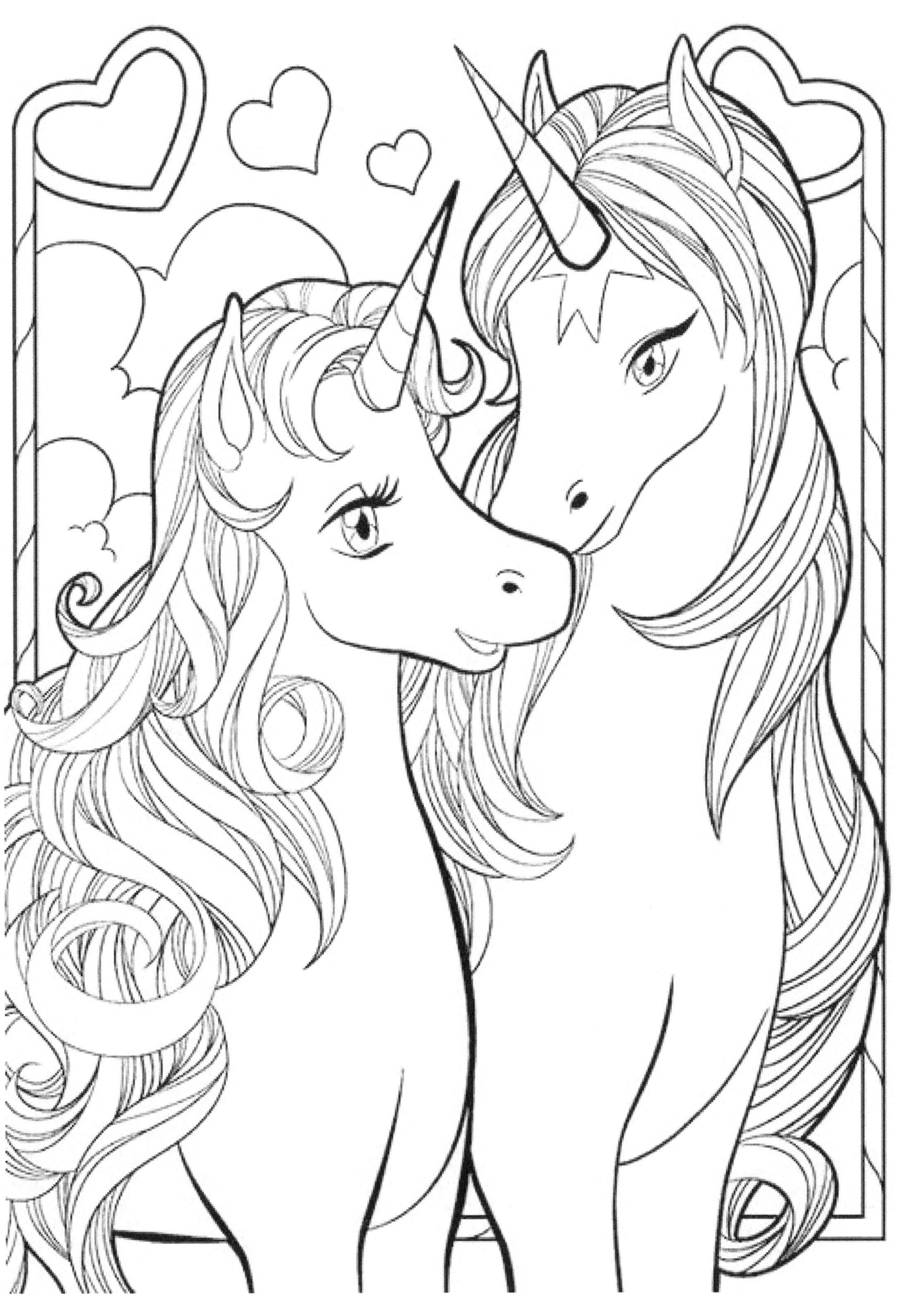

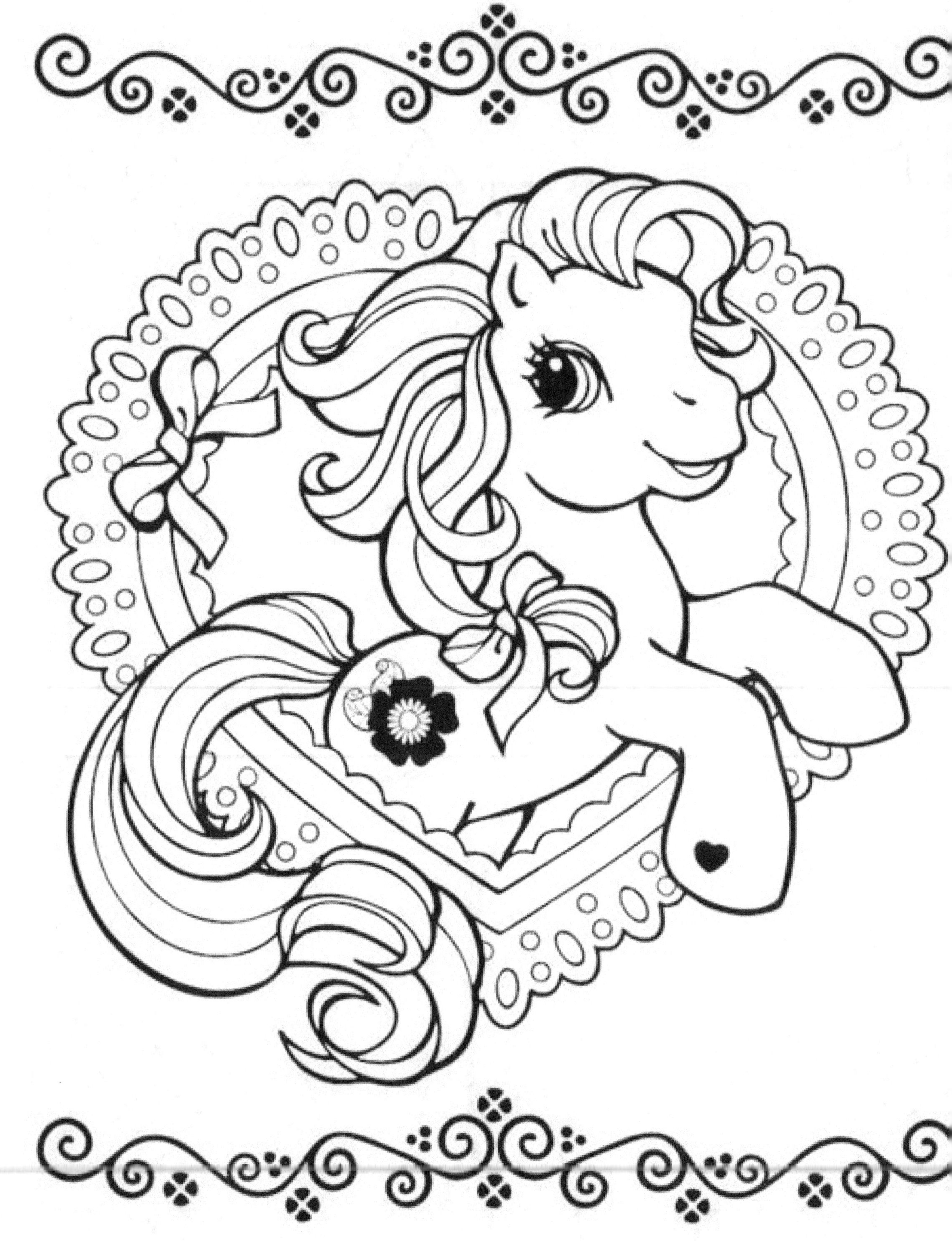

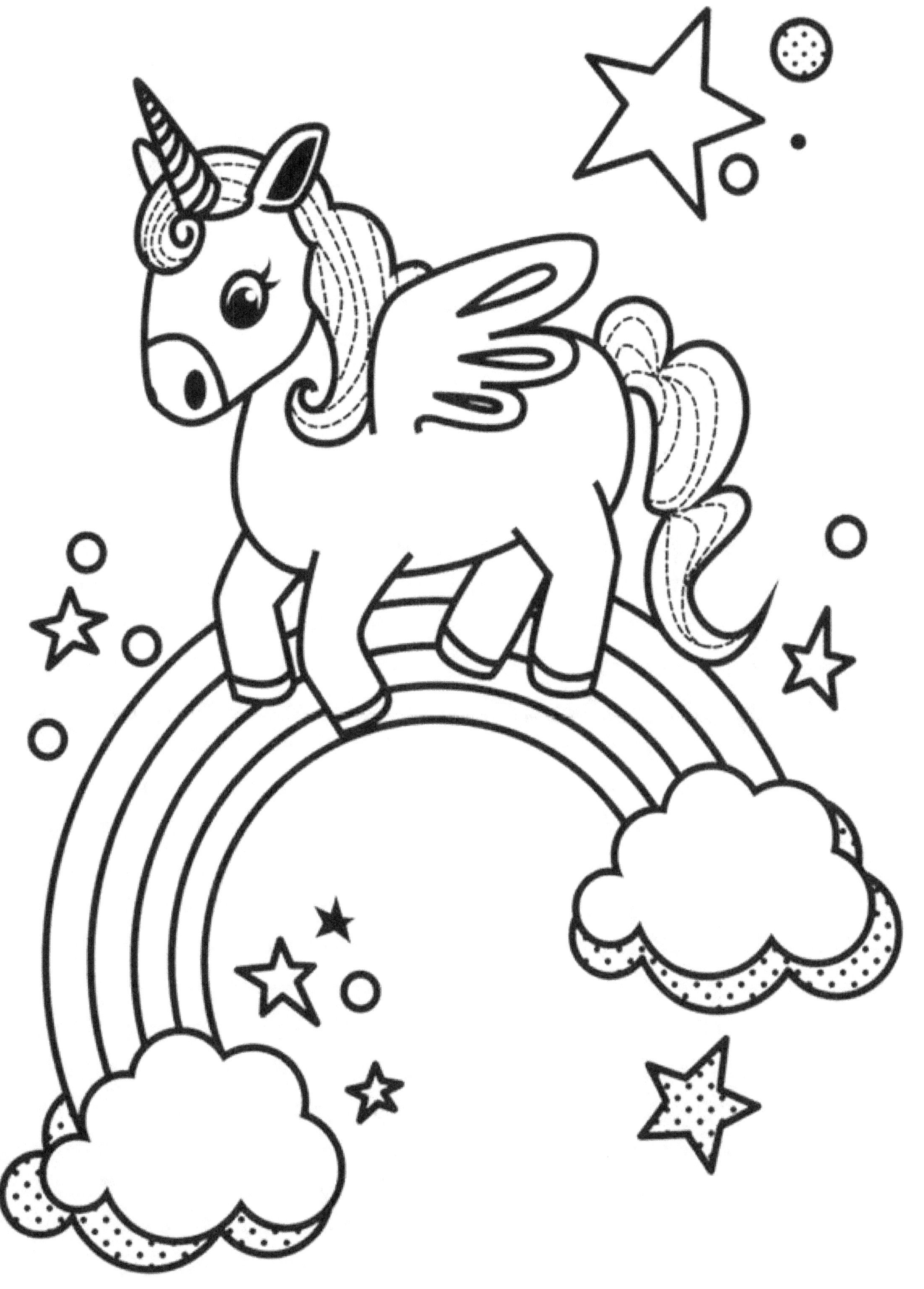

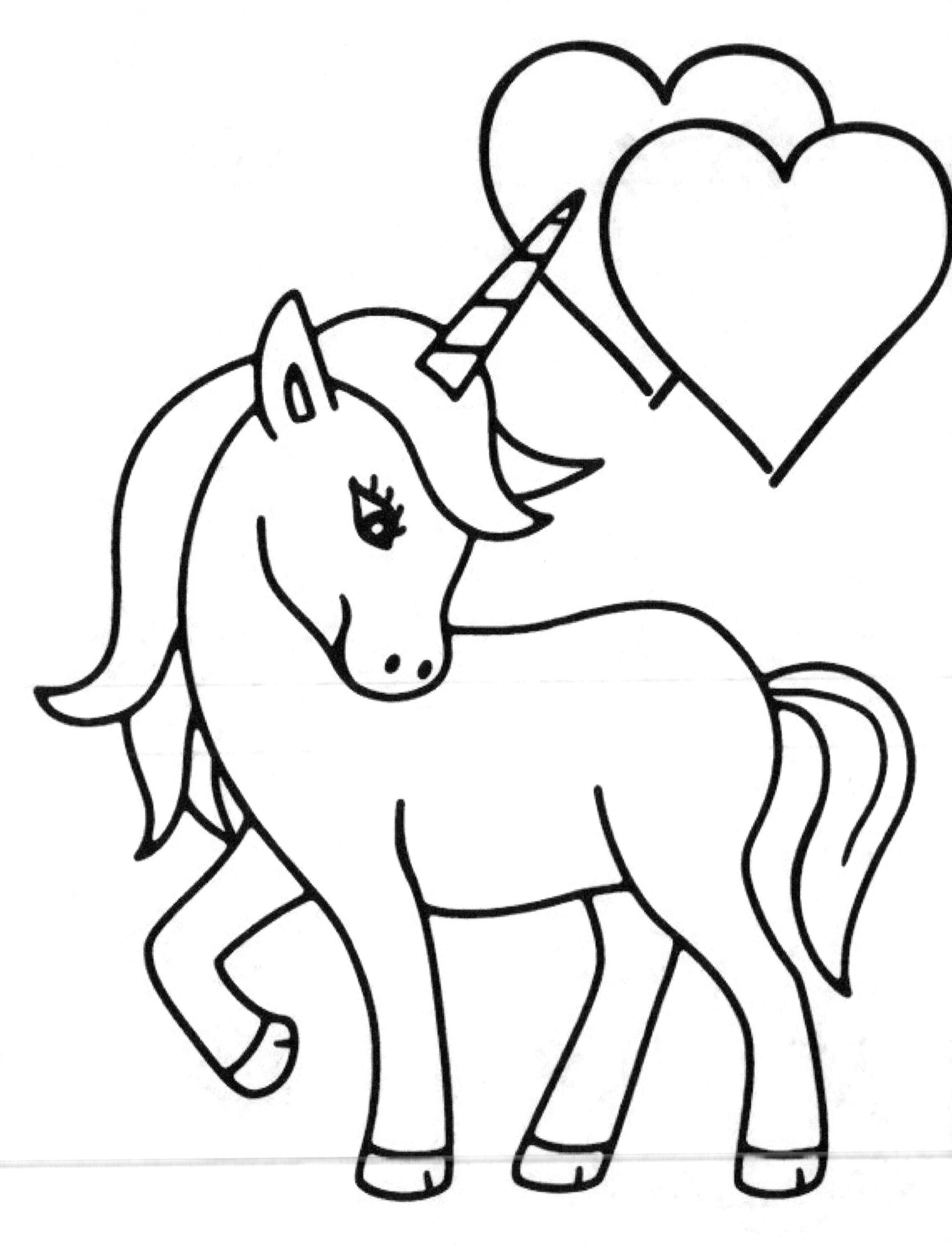

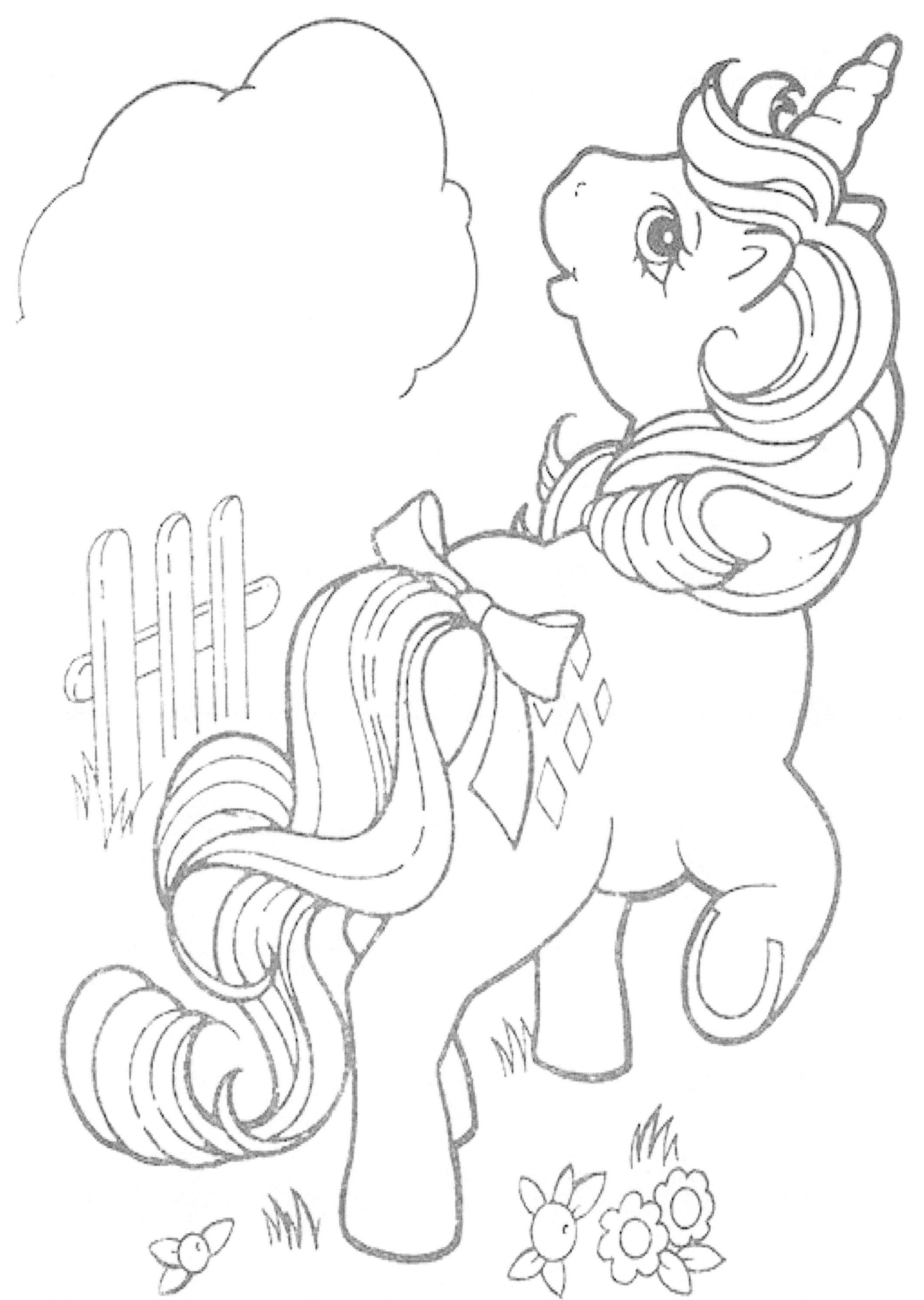

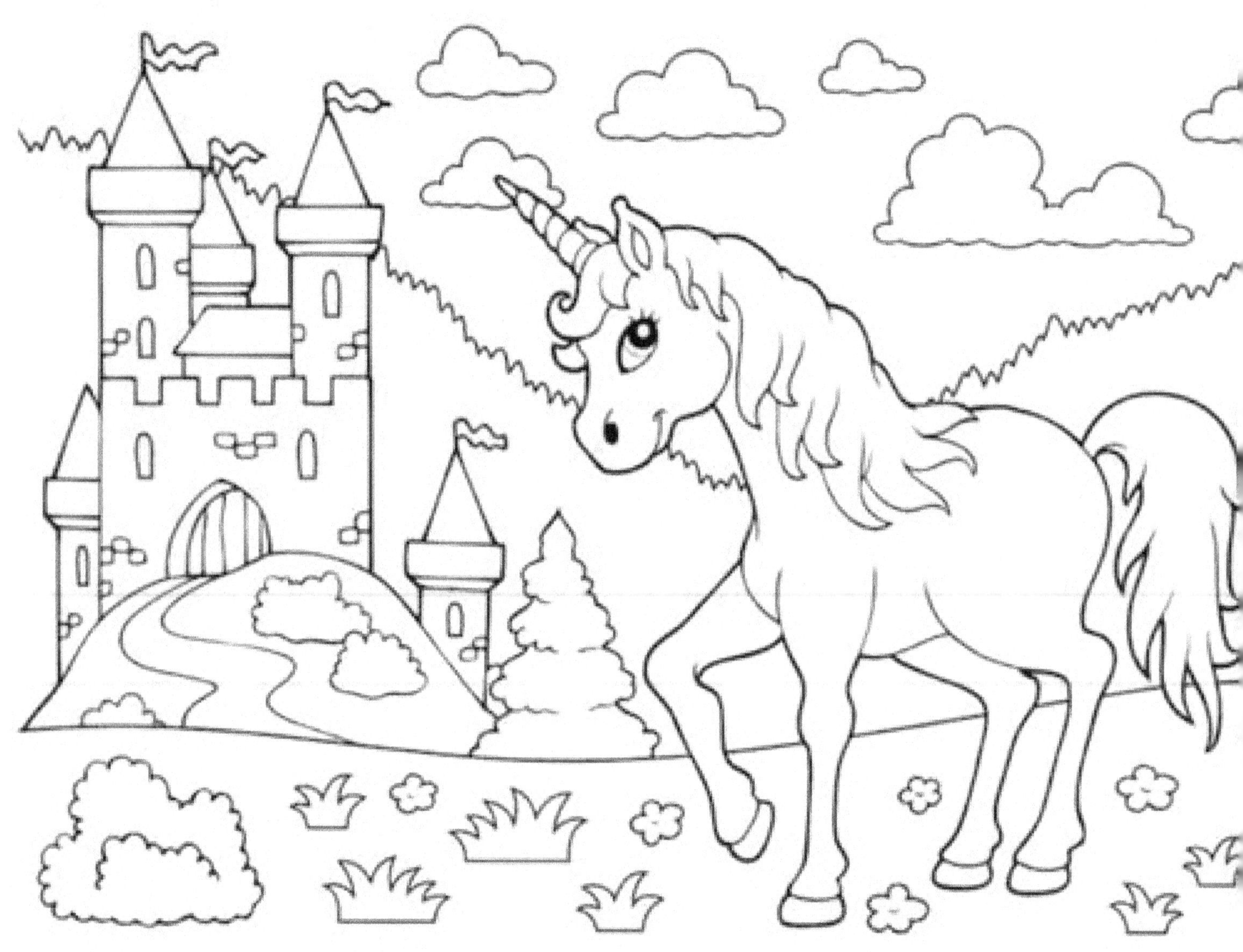

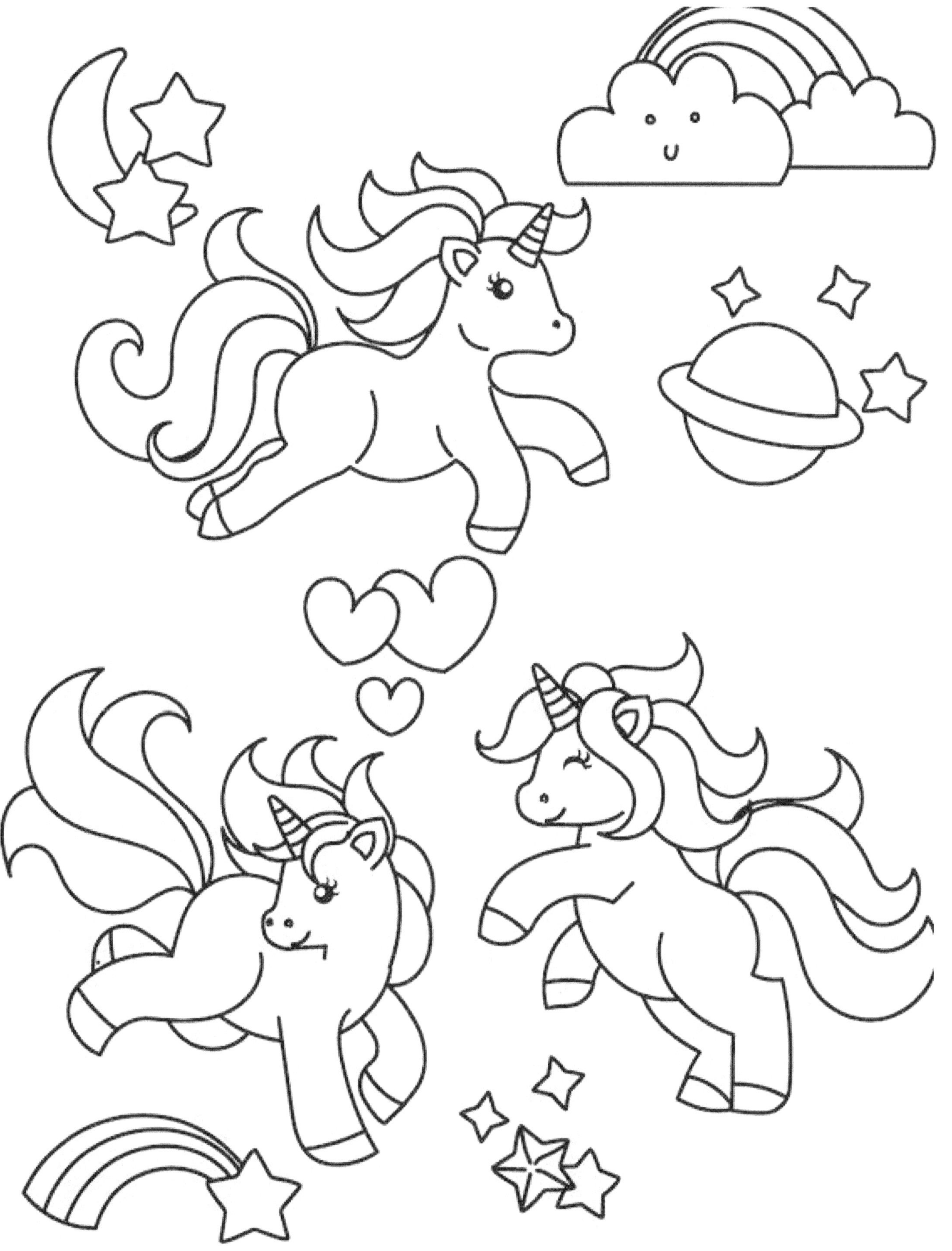

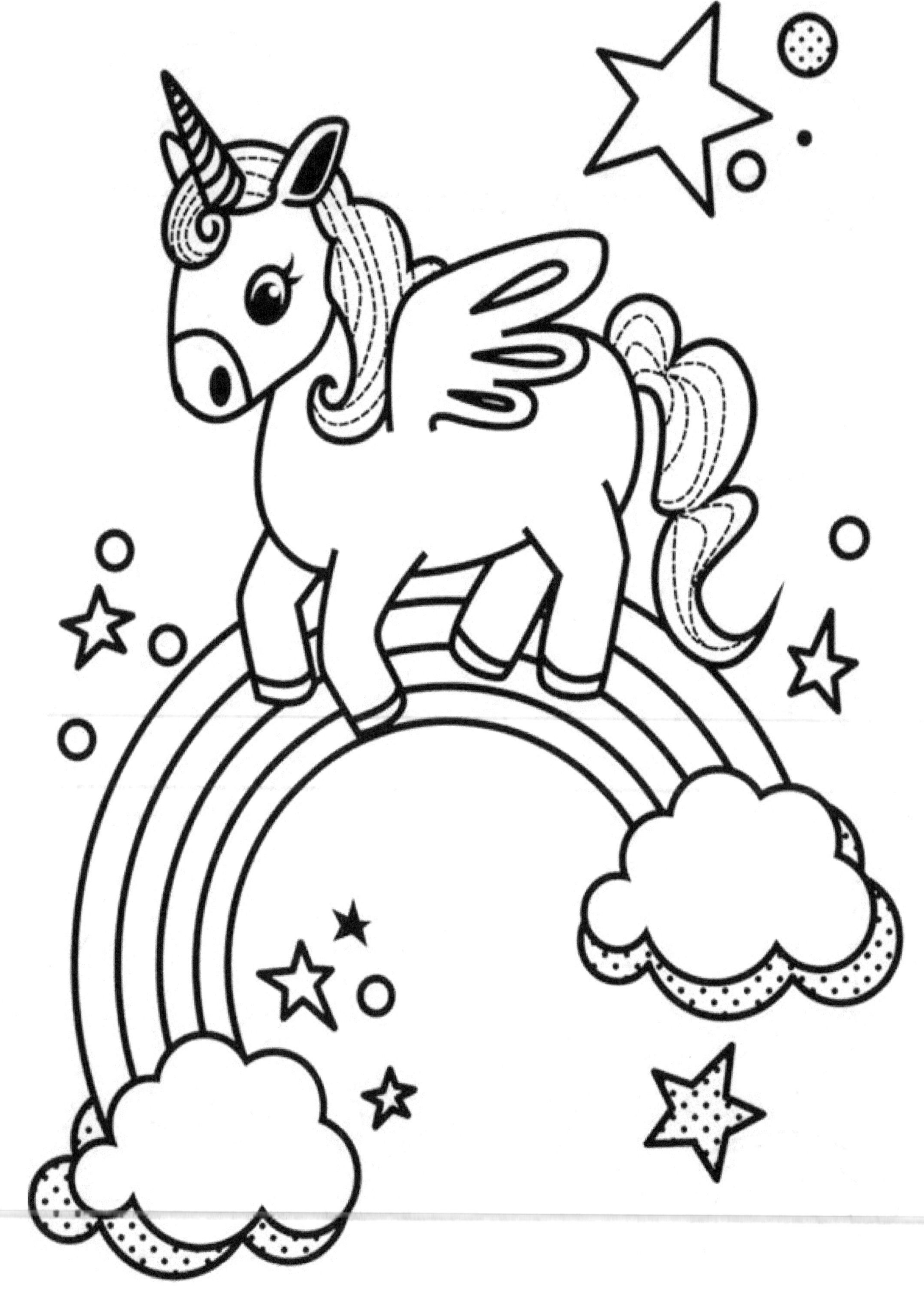

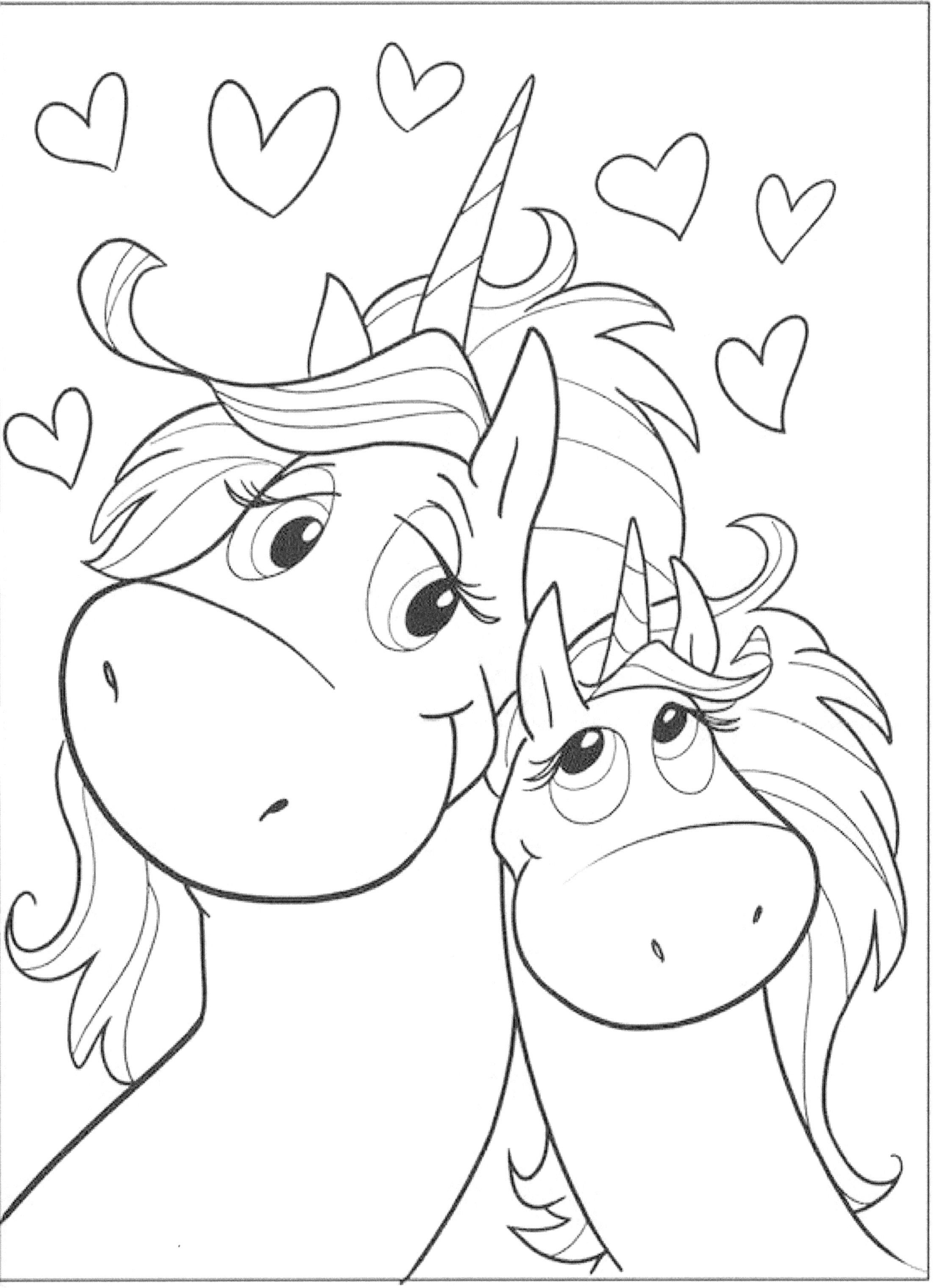

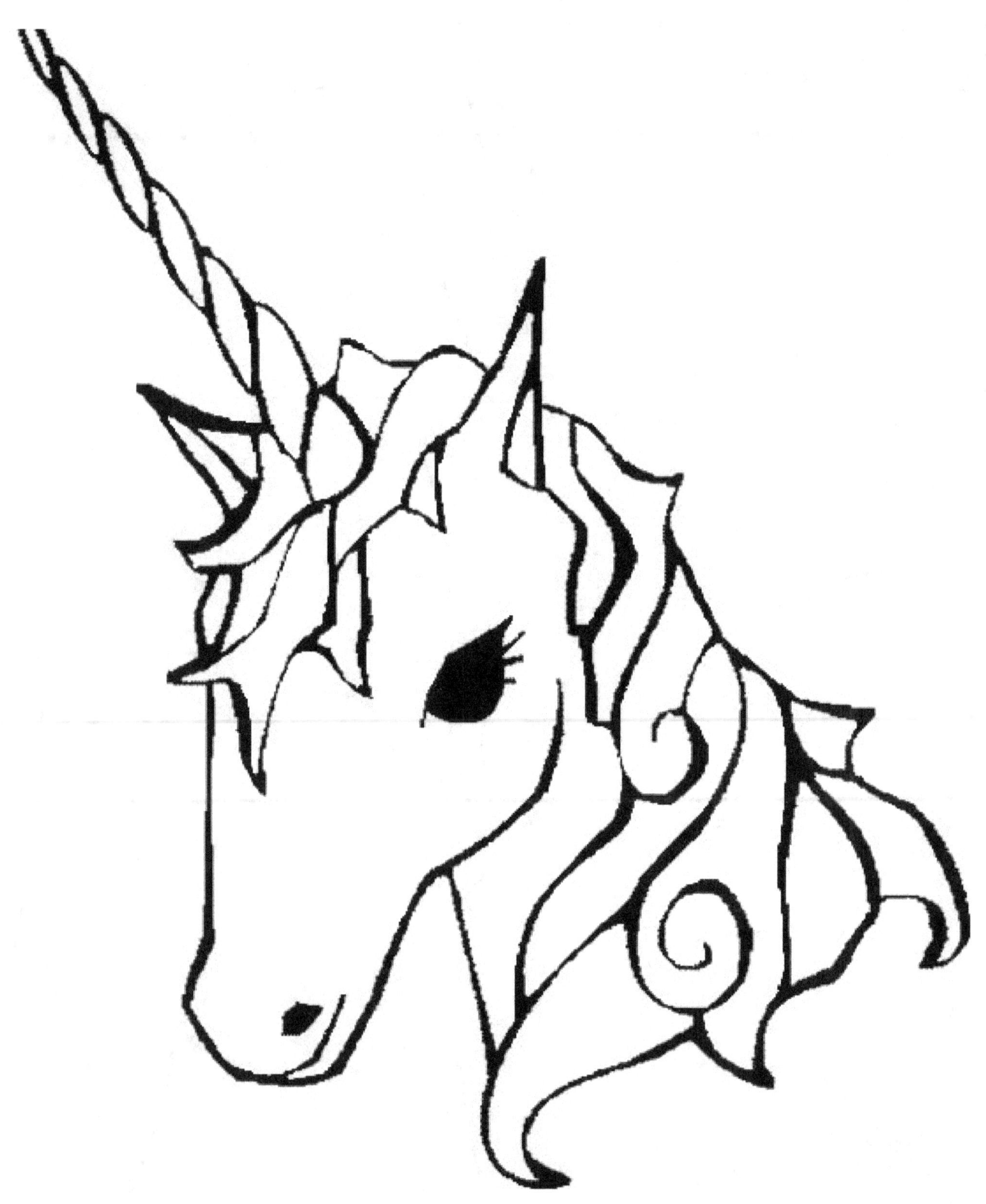

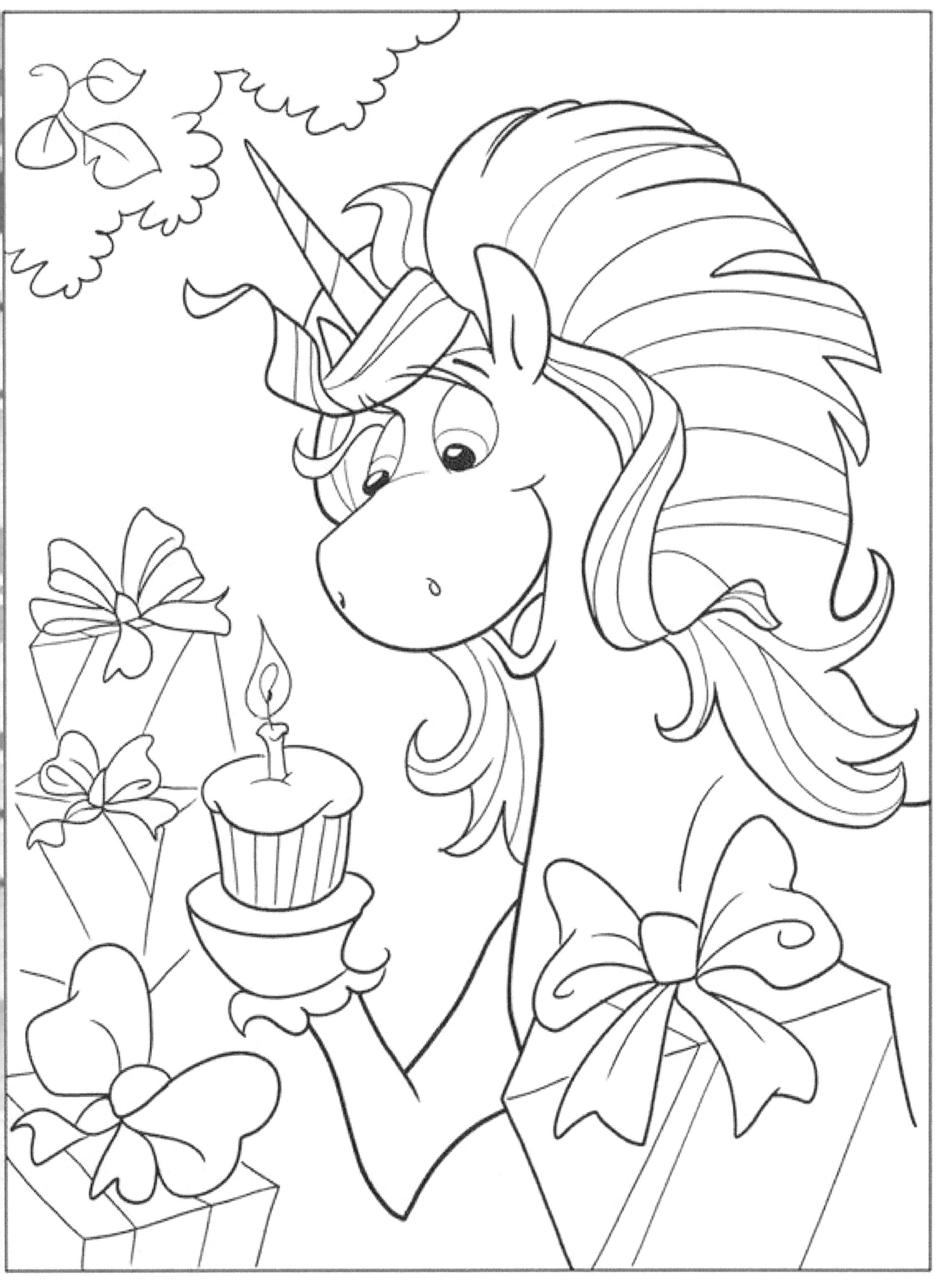

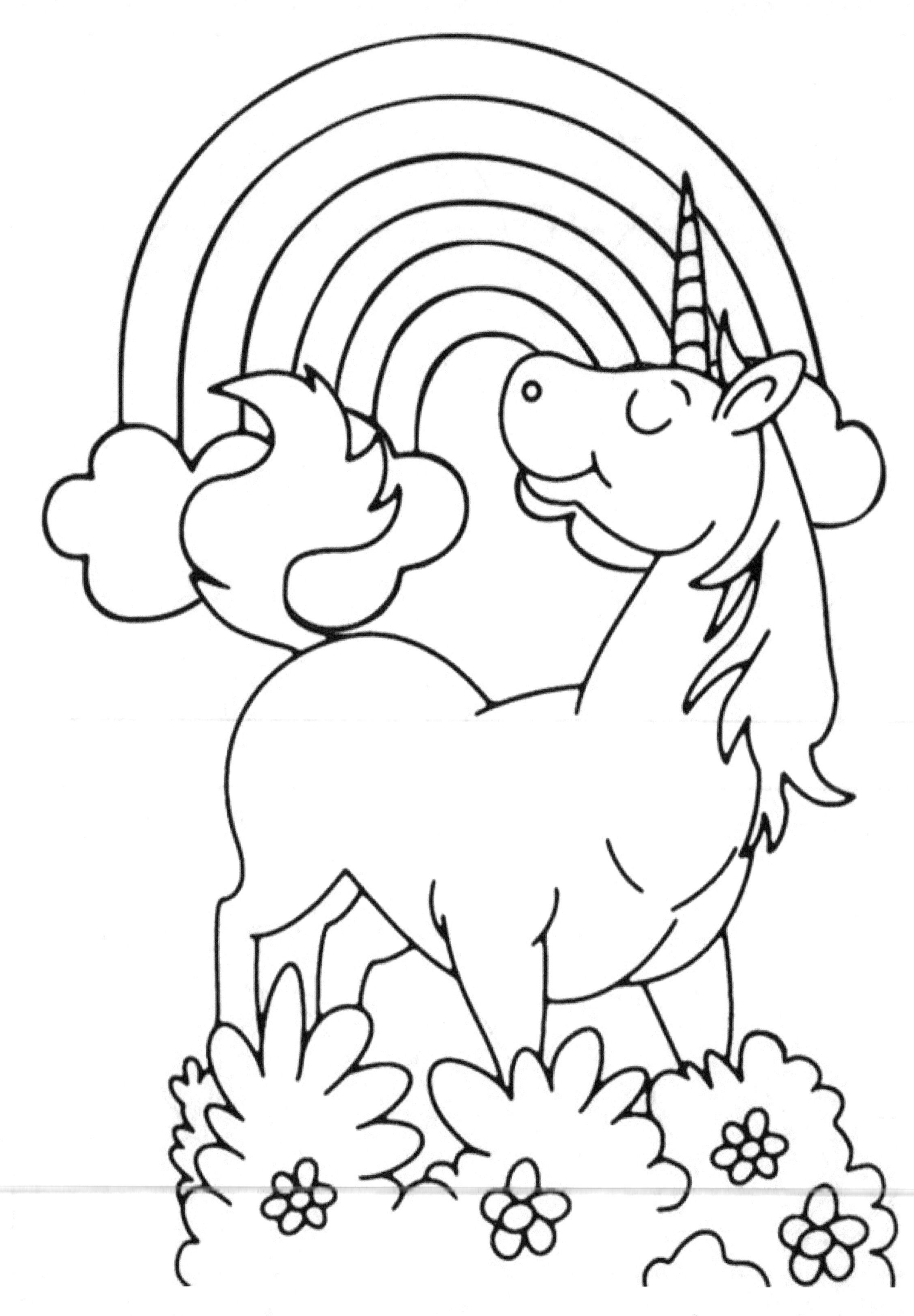

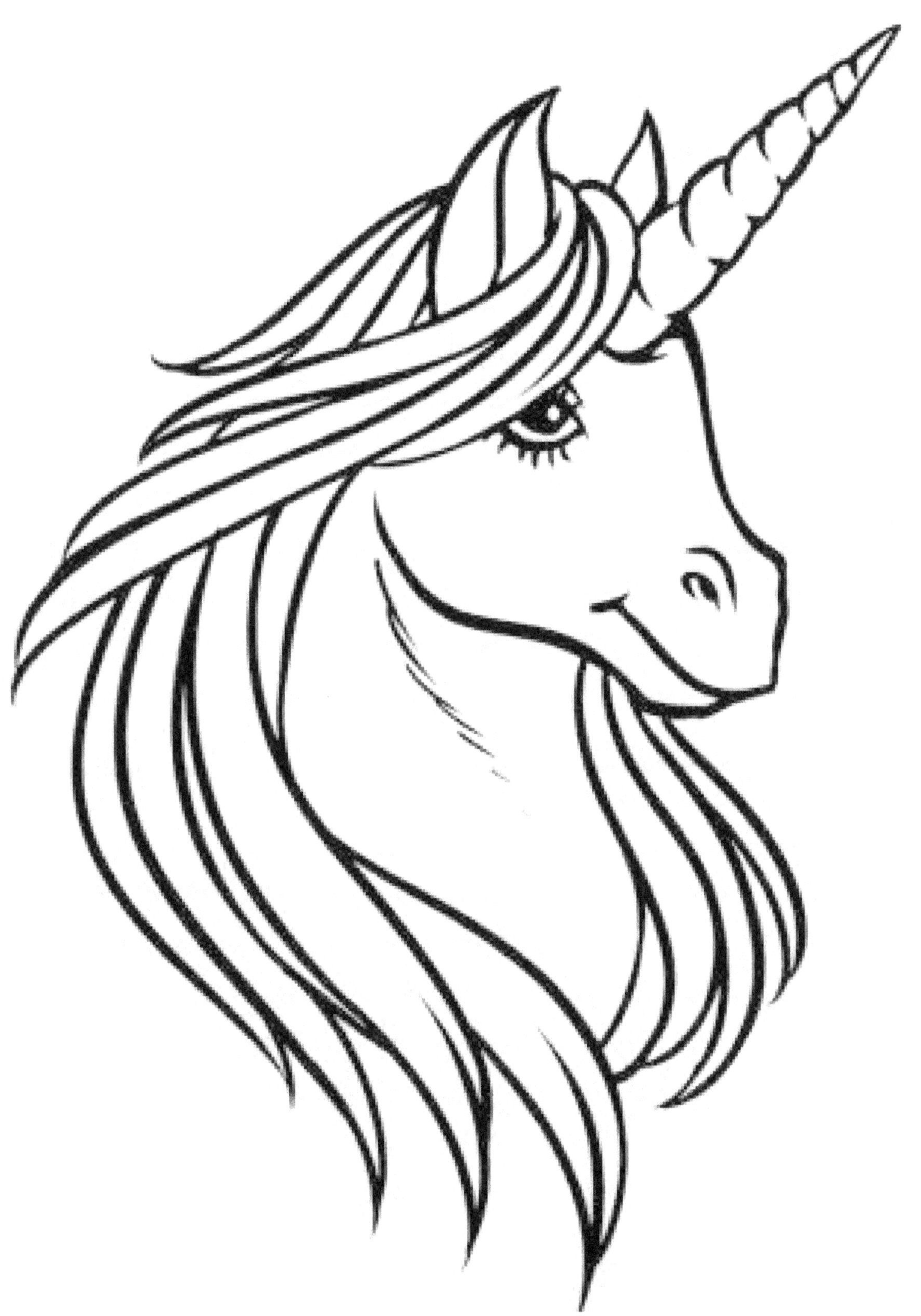

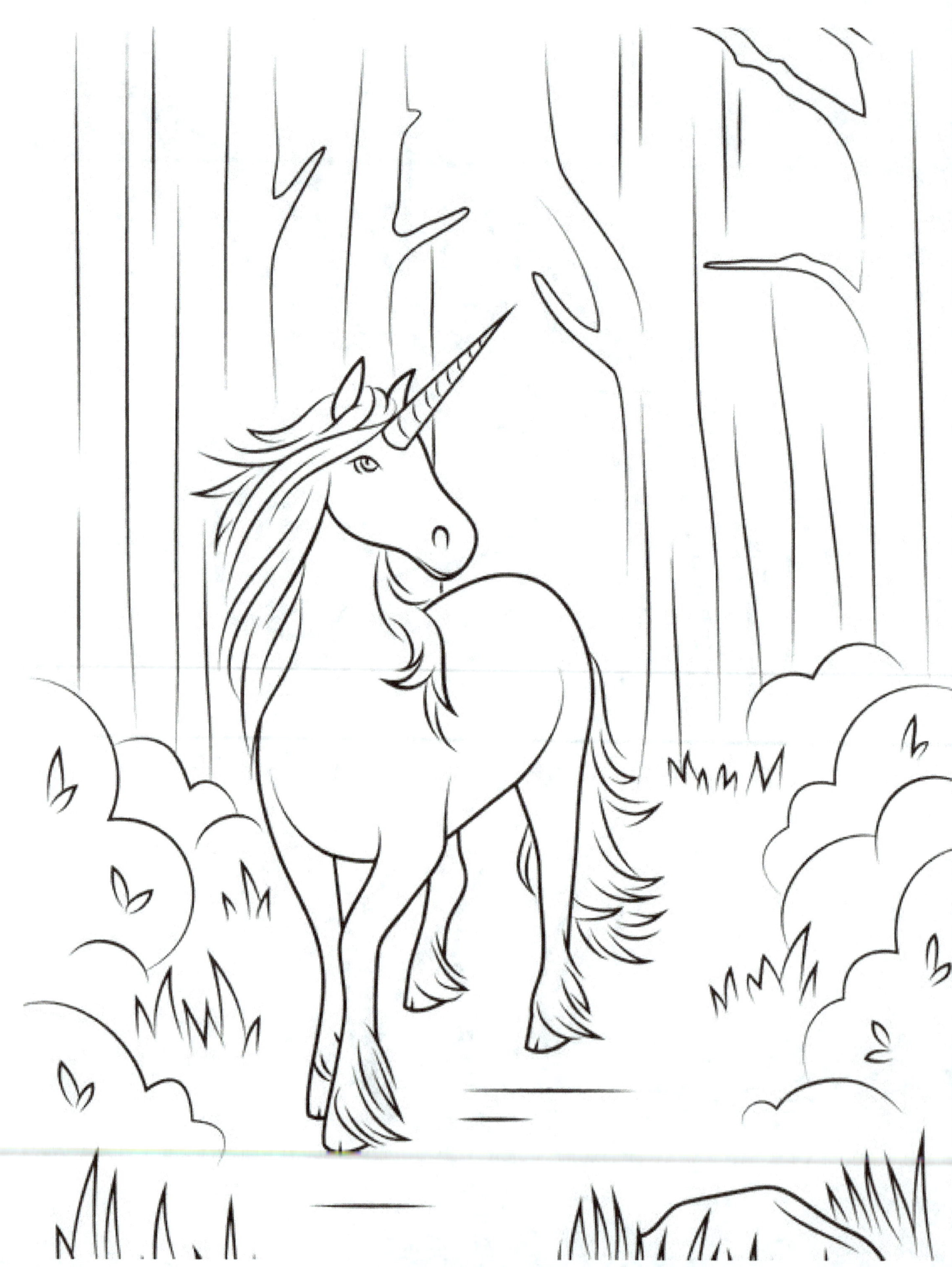

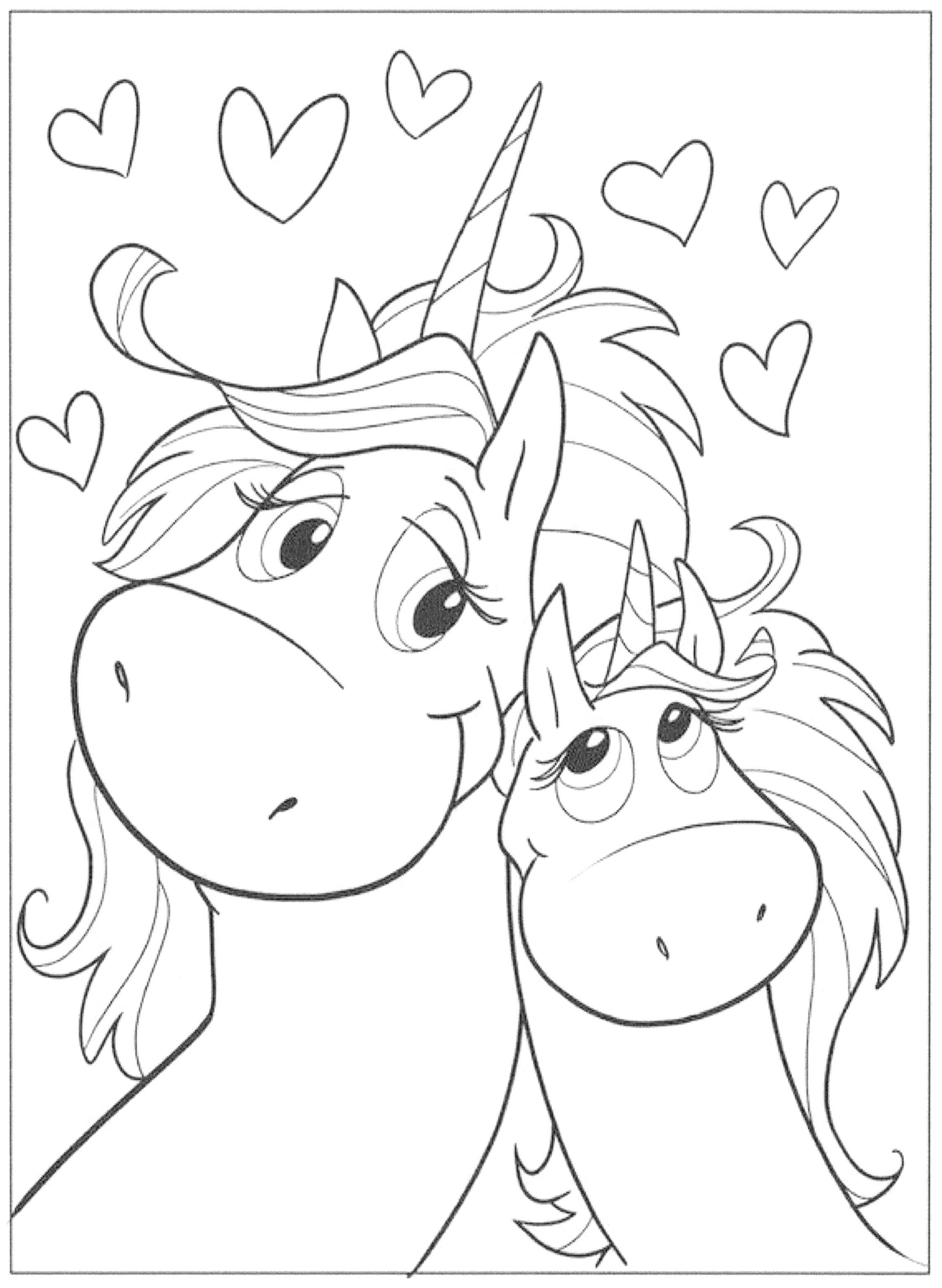

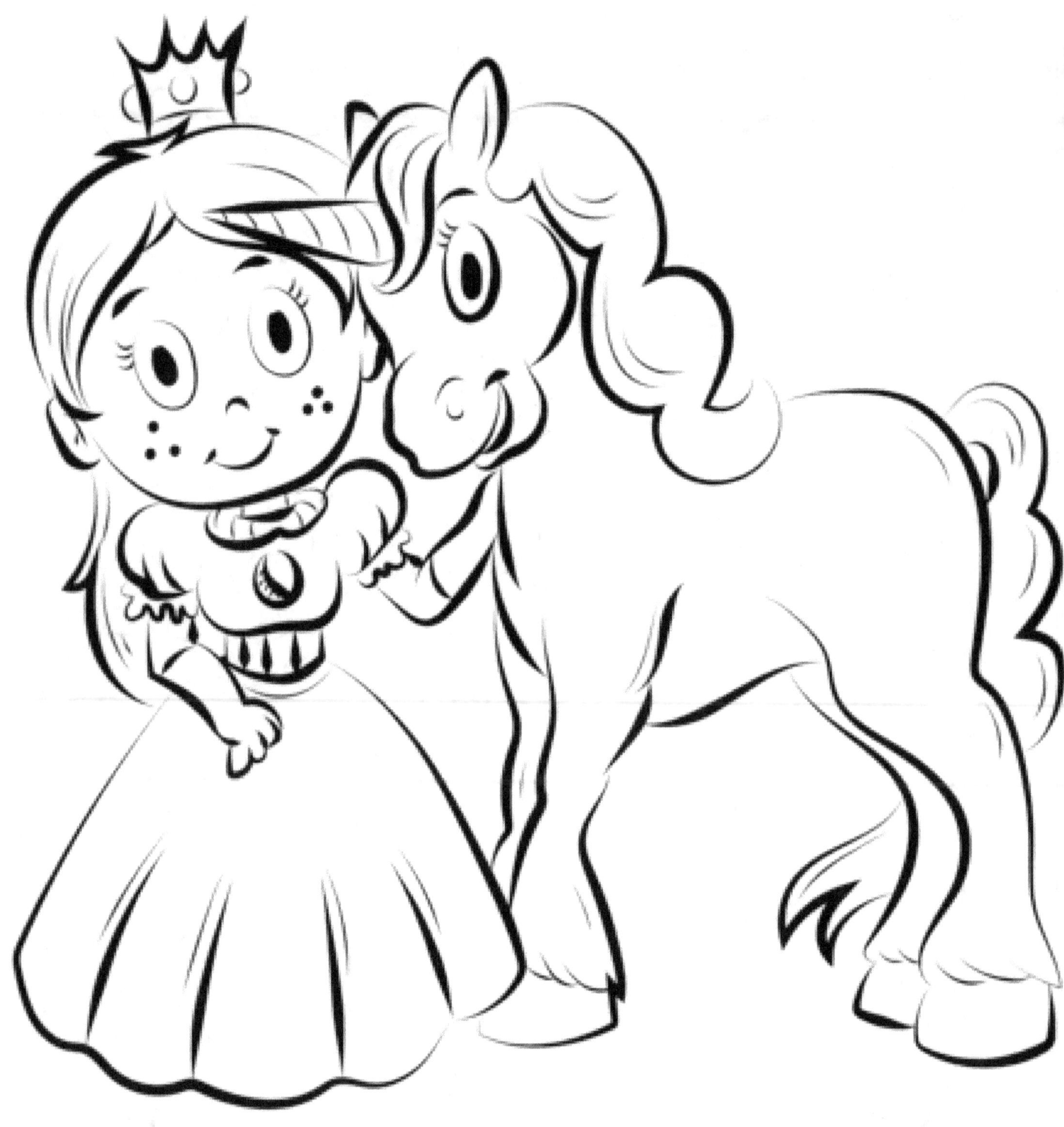

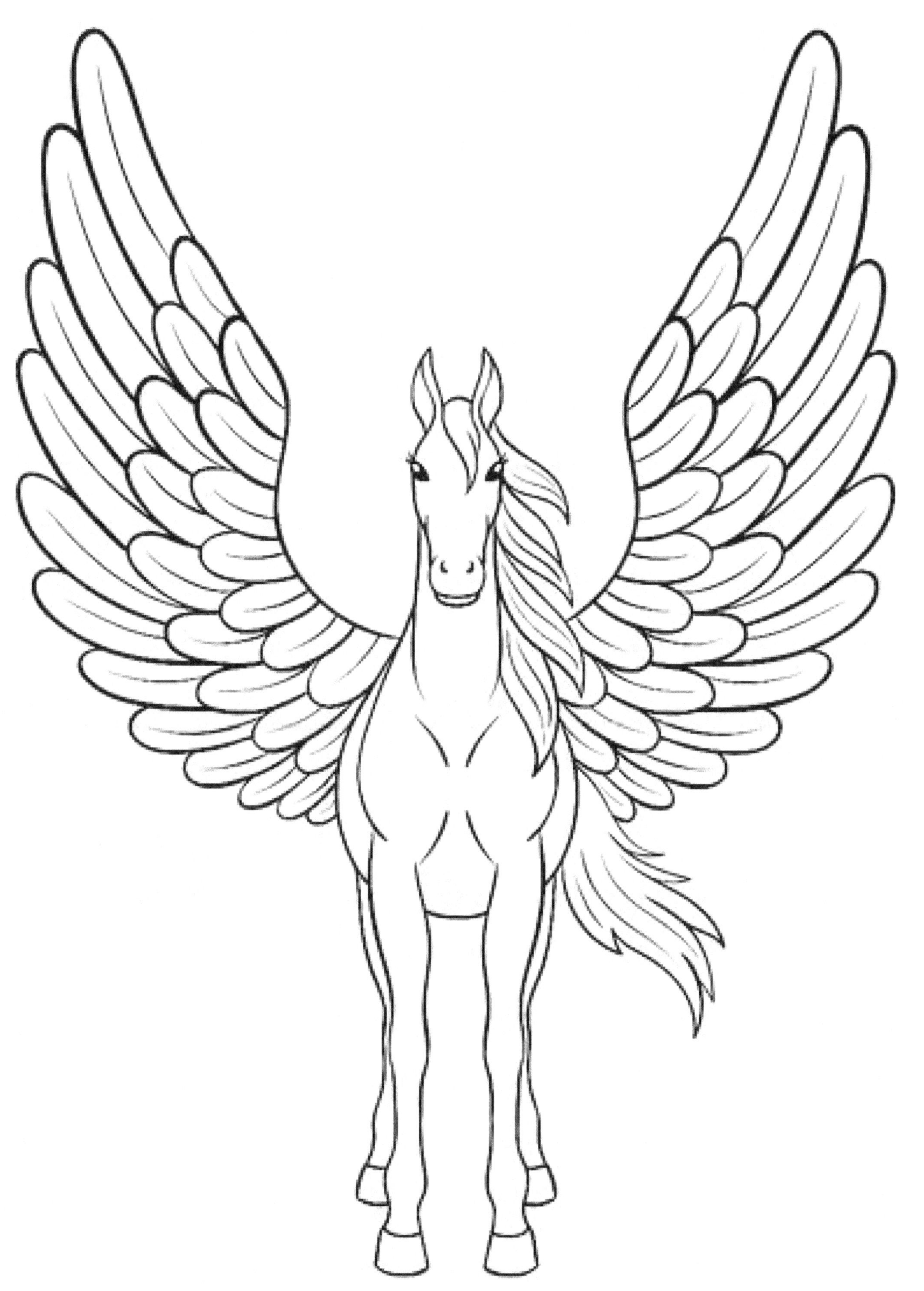

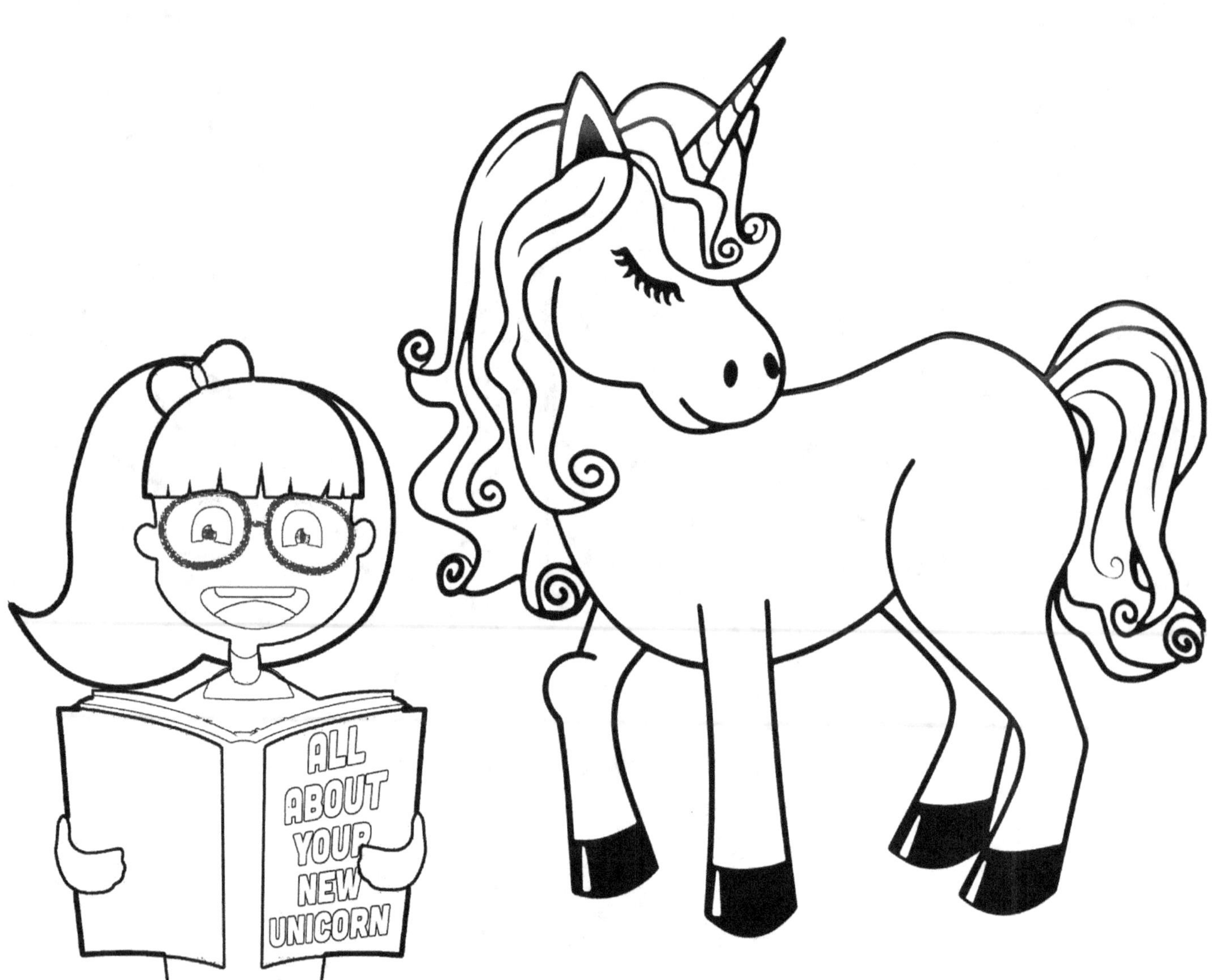

ALL
ABOUT
YOUR
NEW
UNICORN

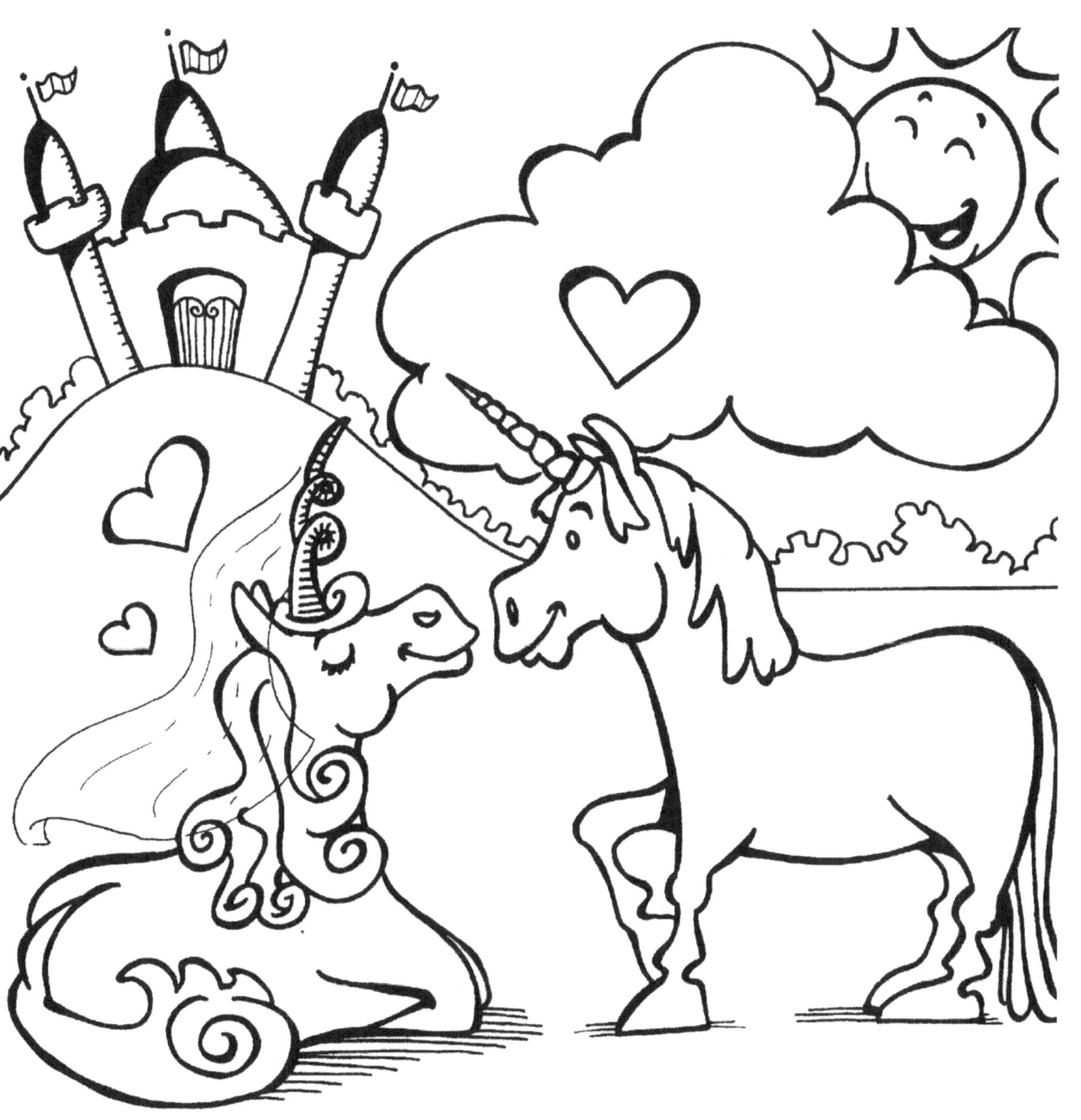

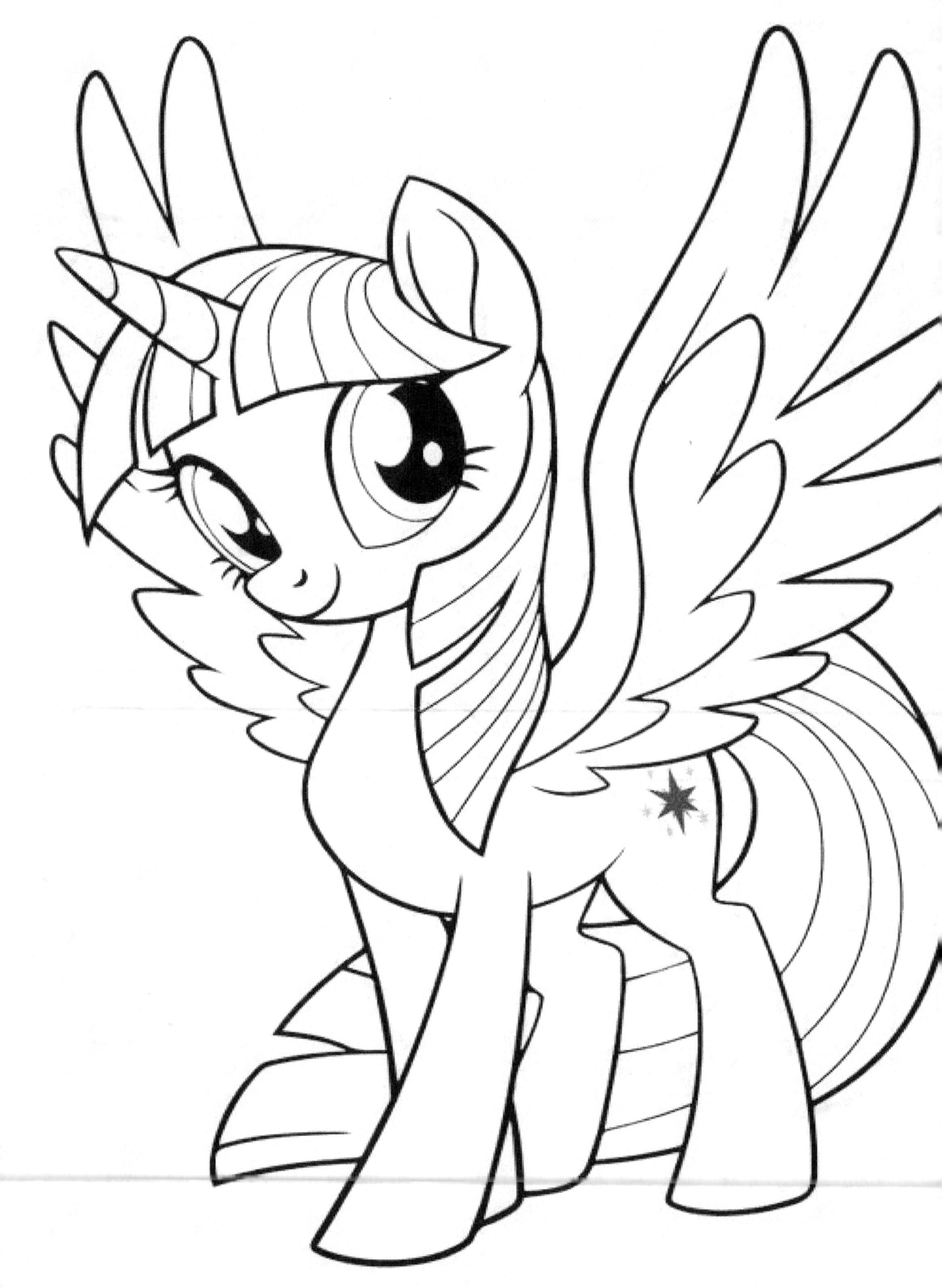

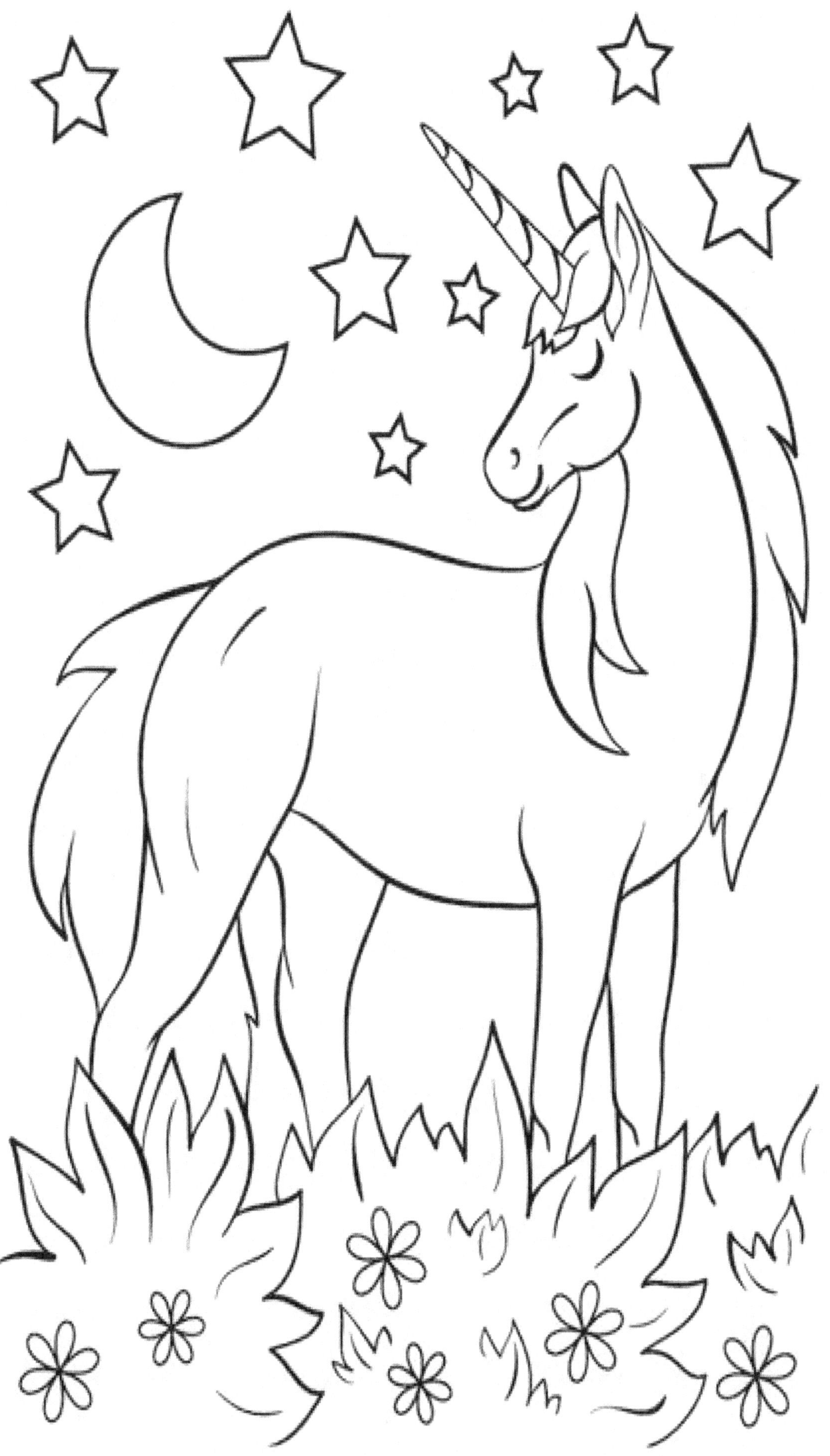

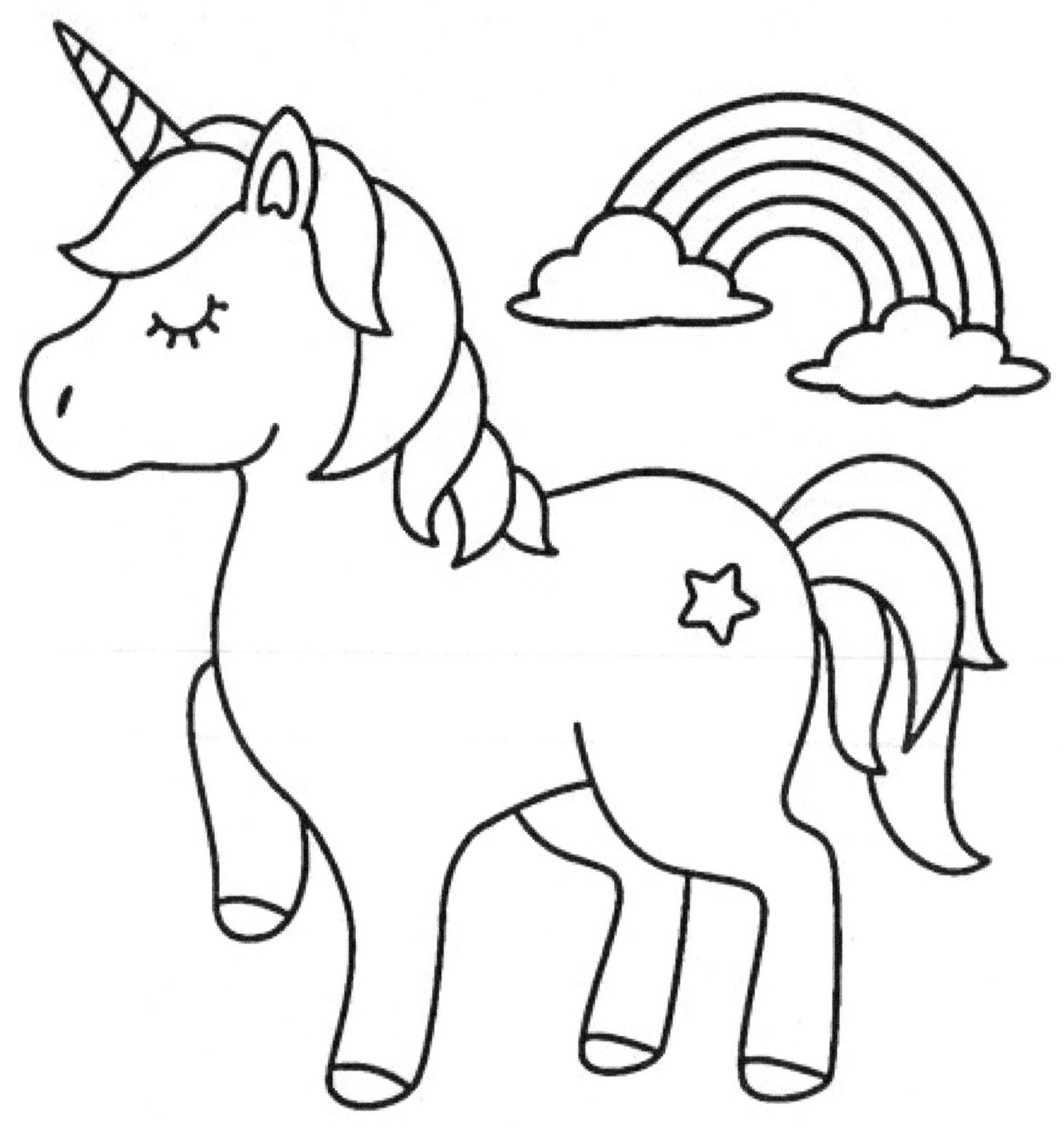

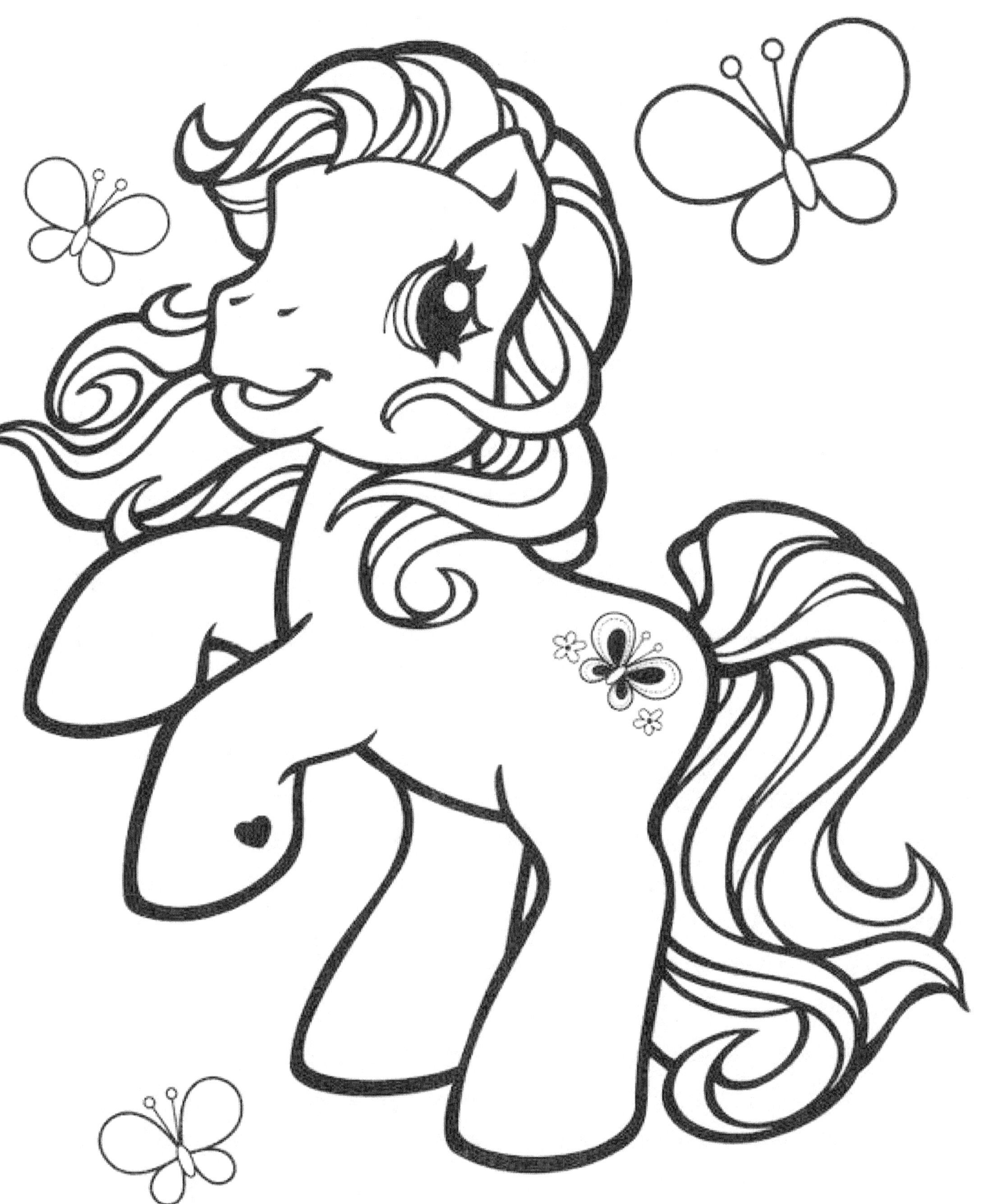

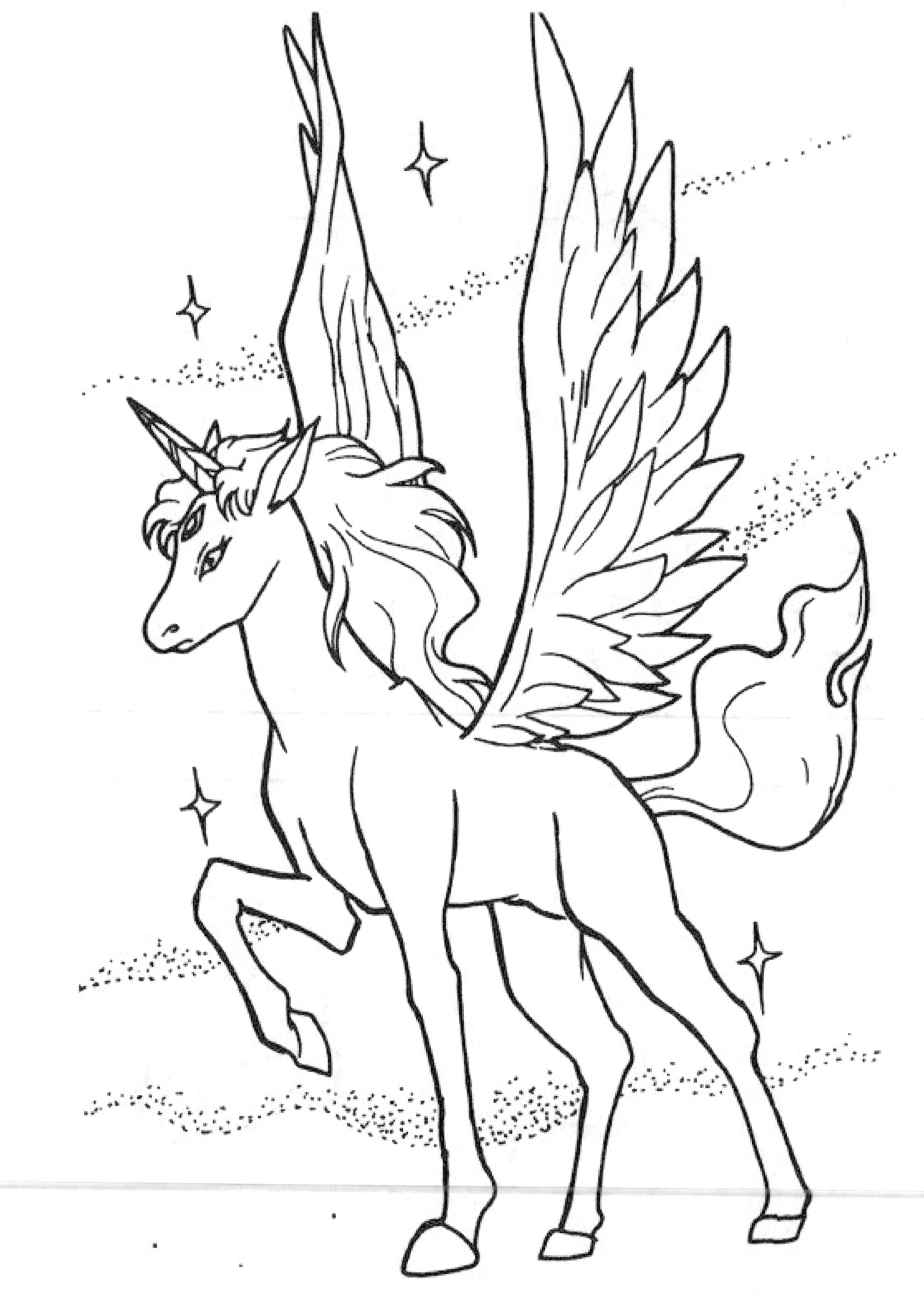

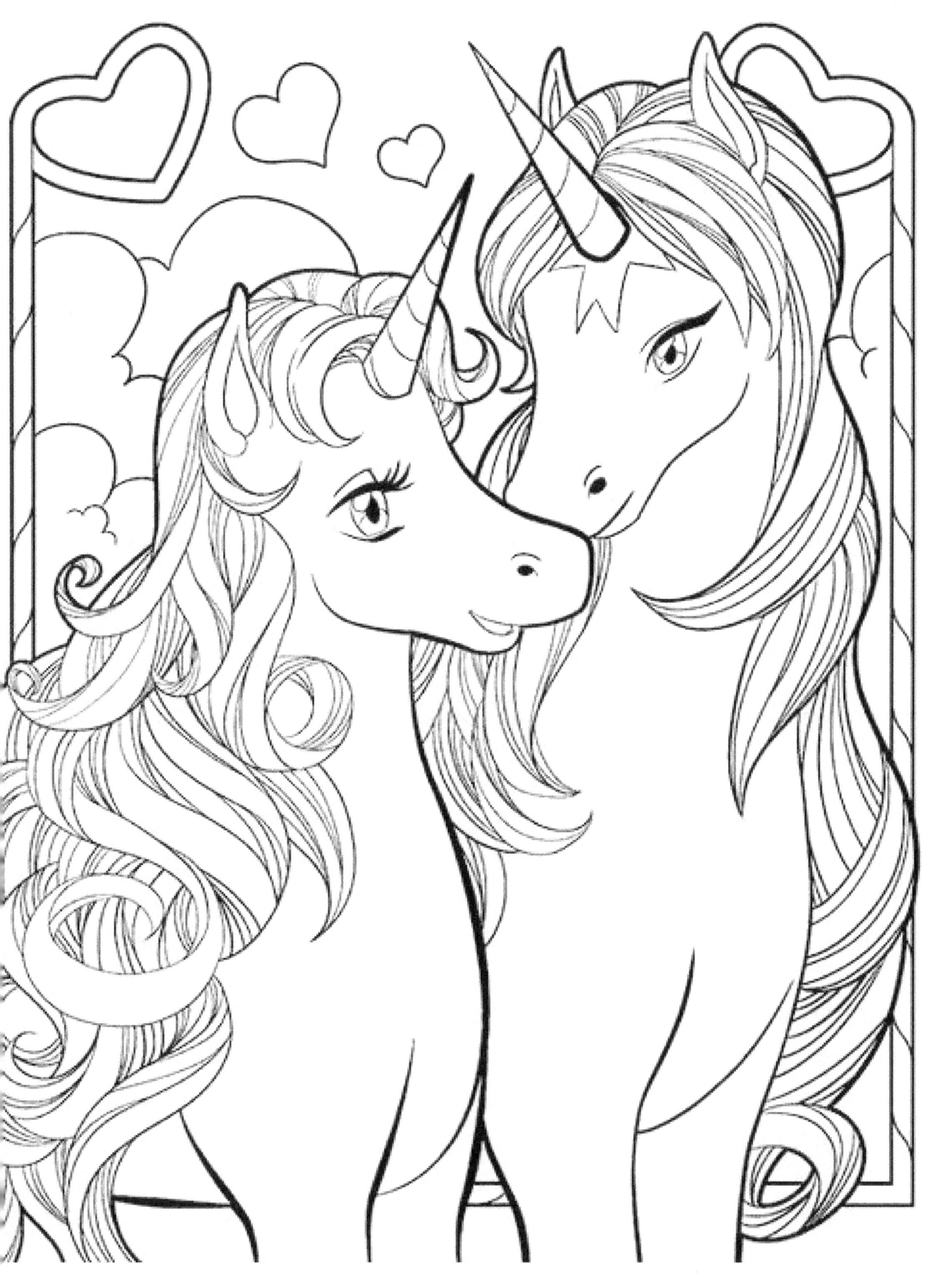

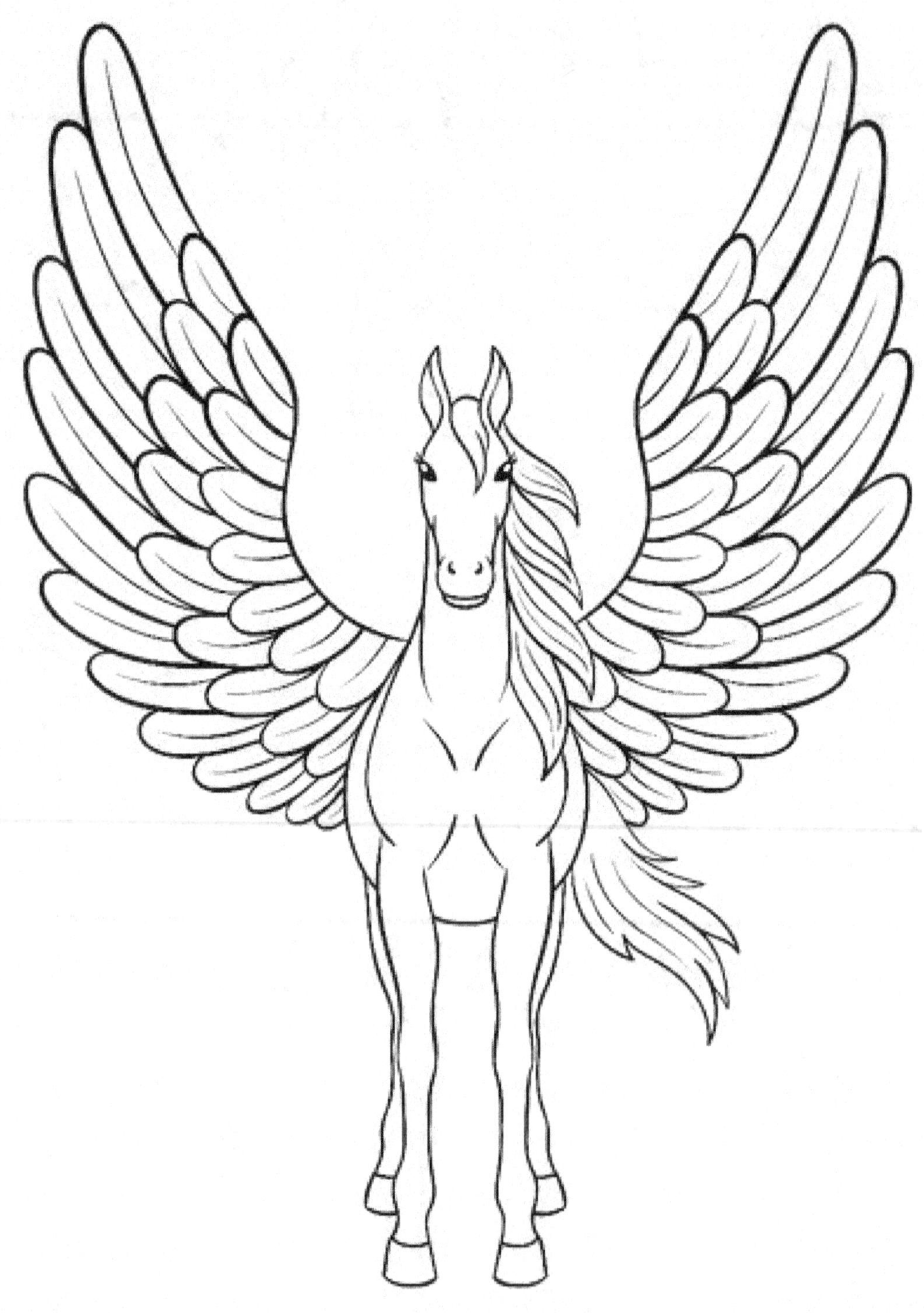

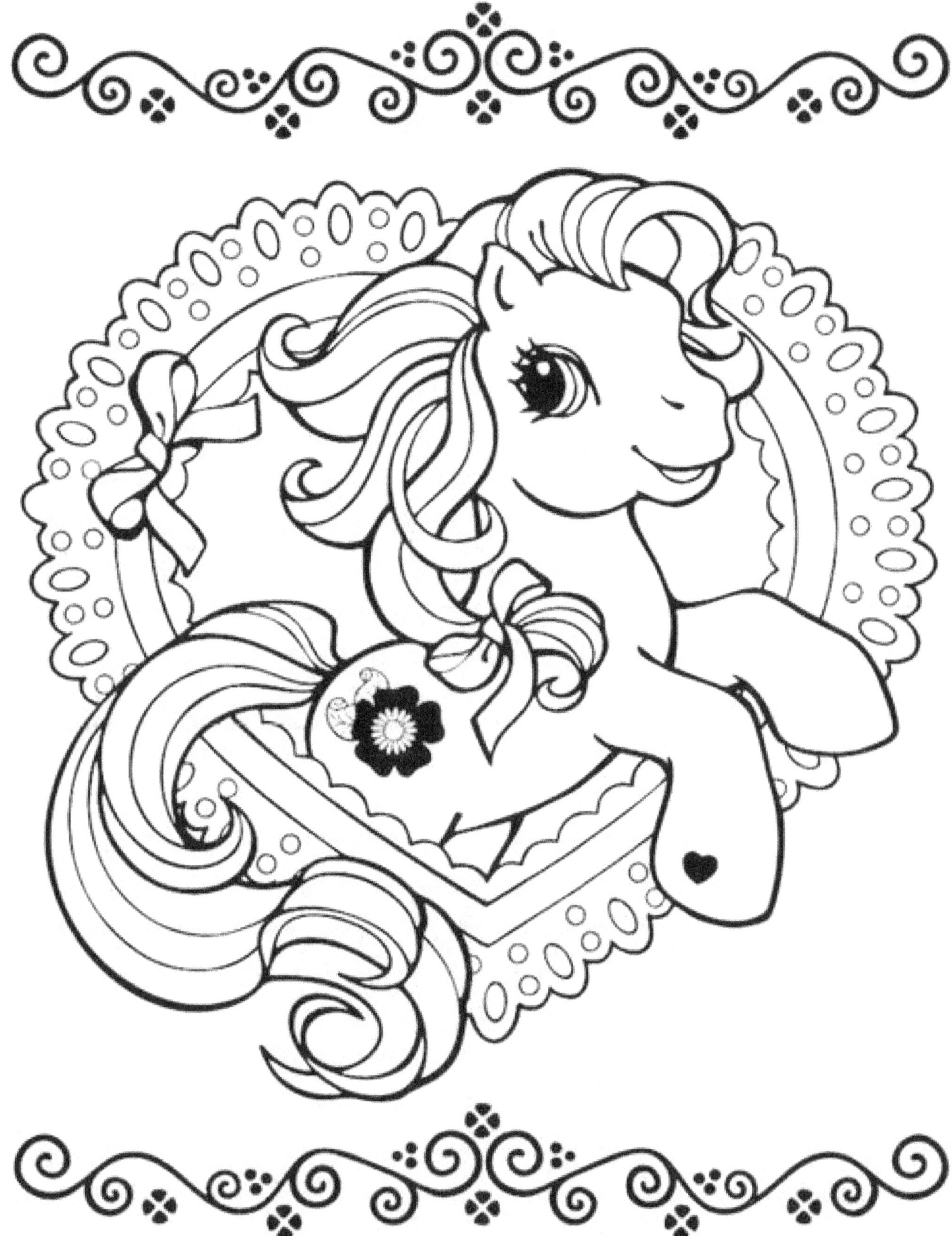

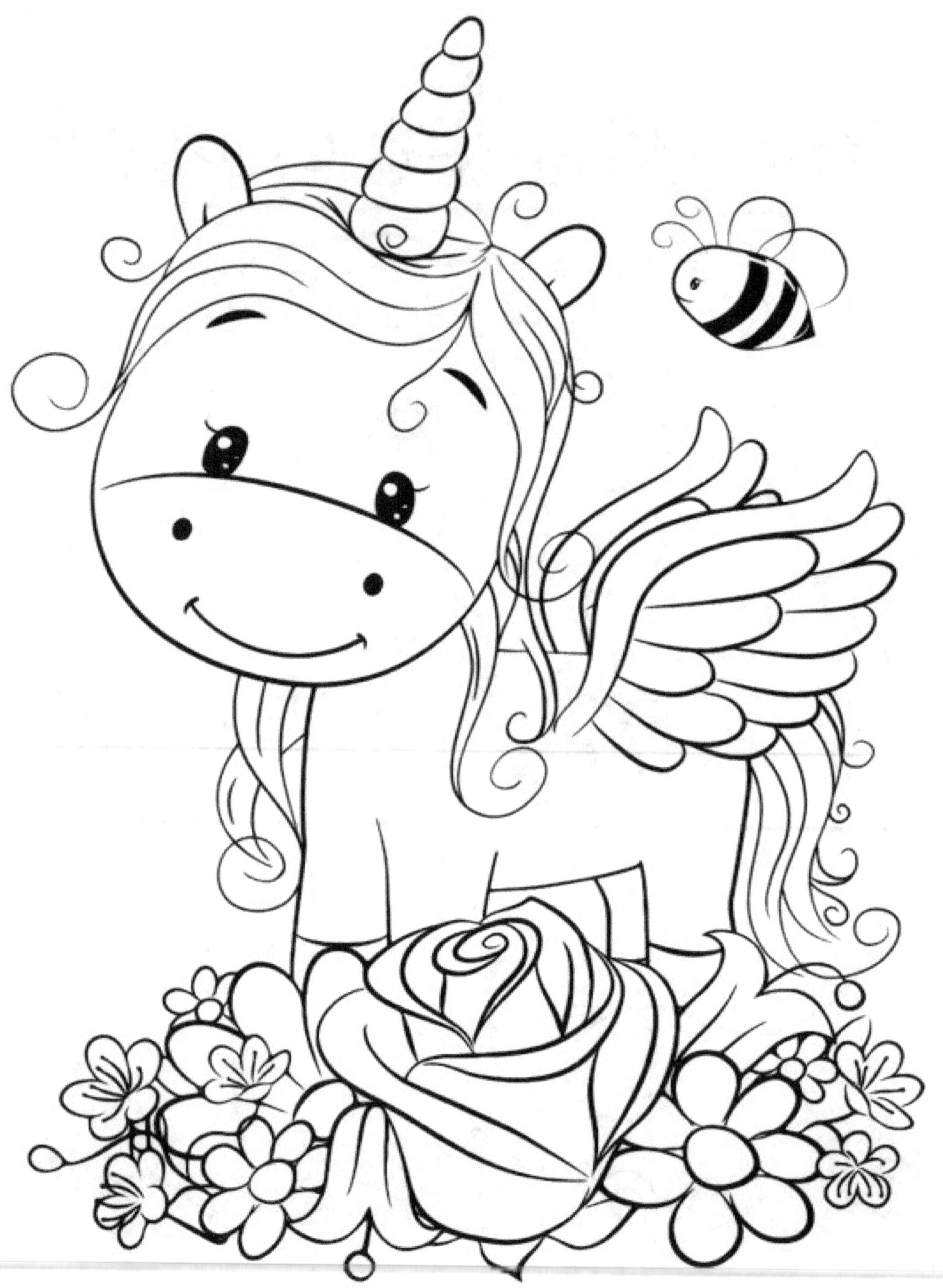

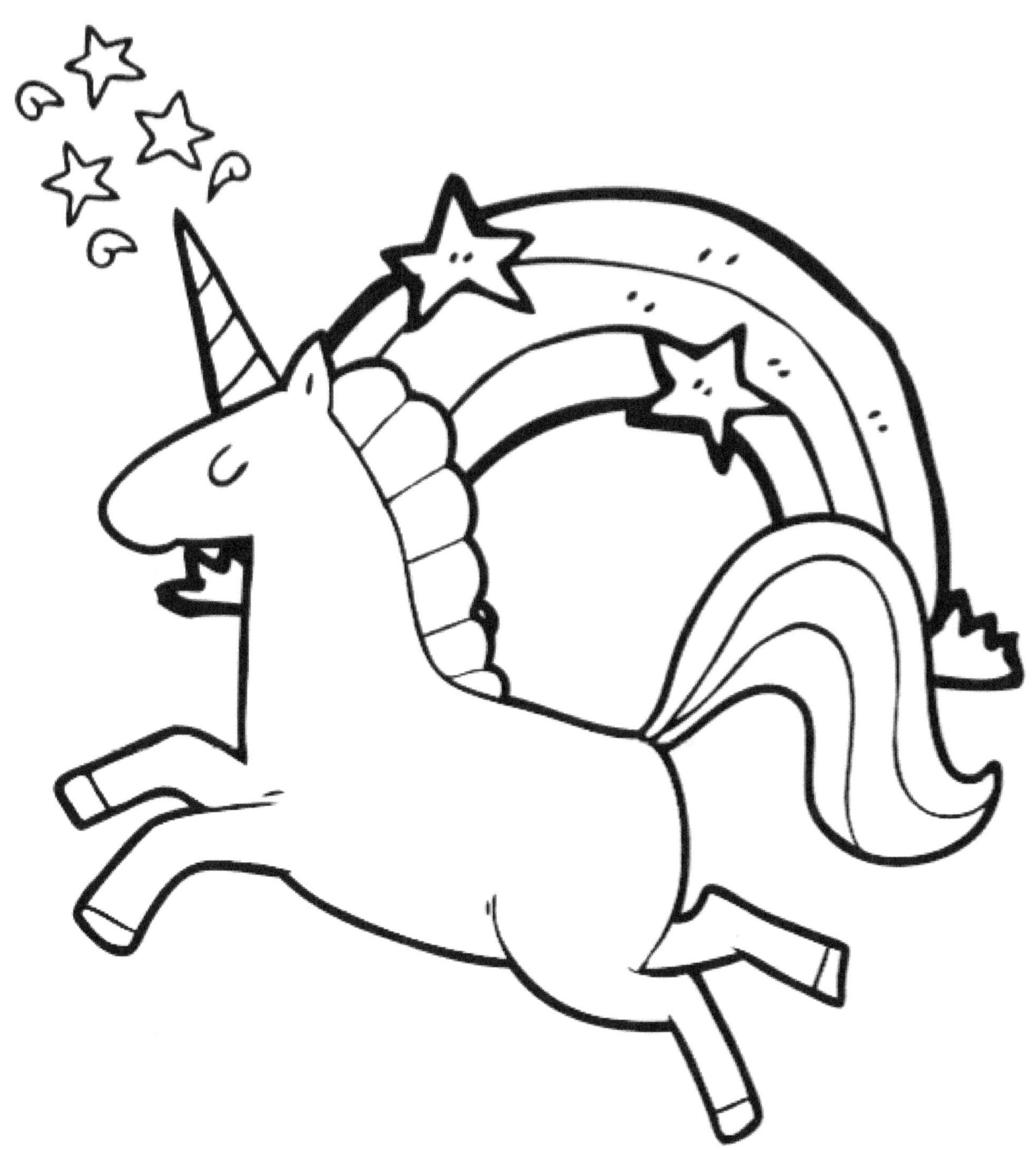

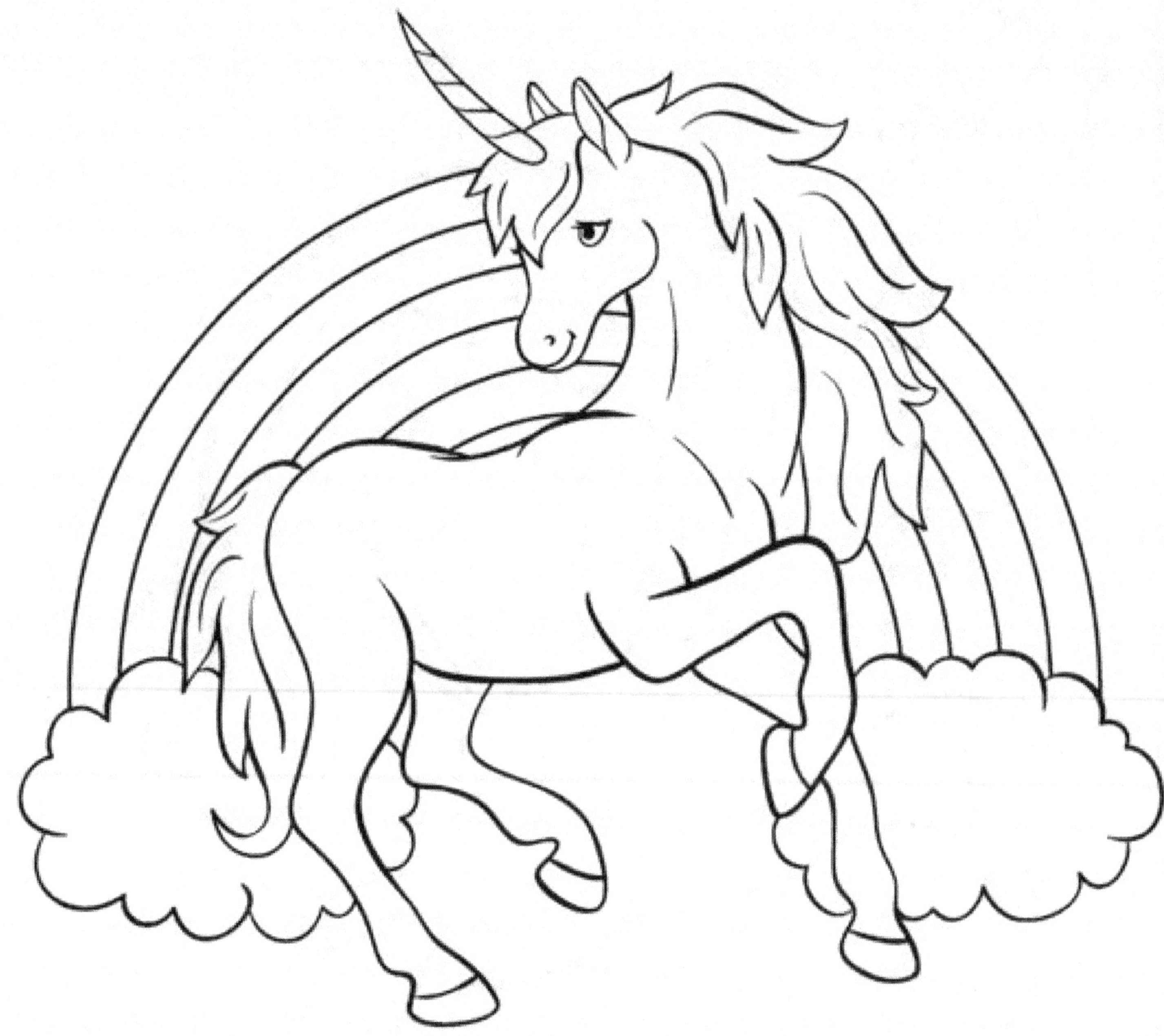

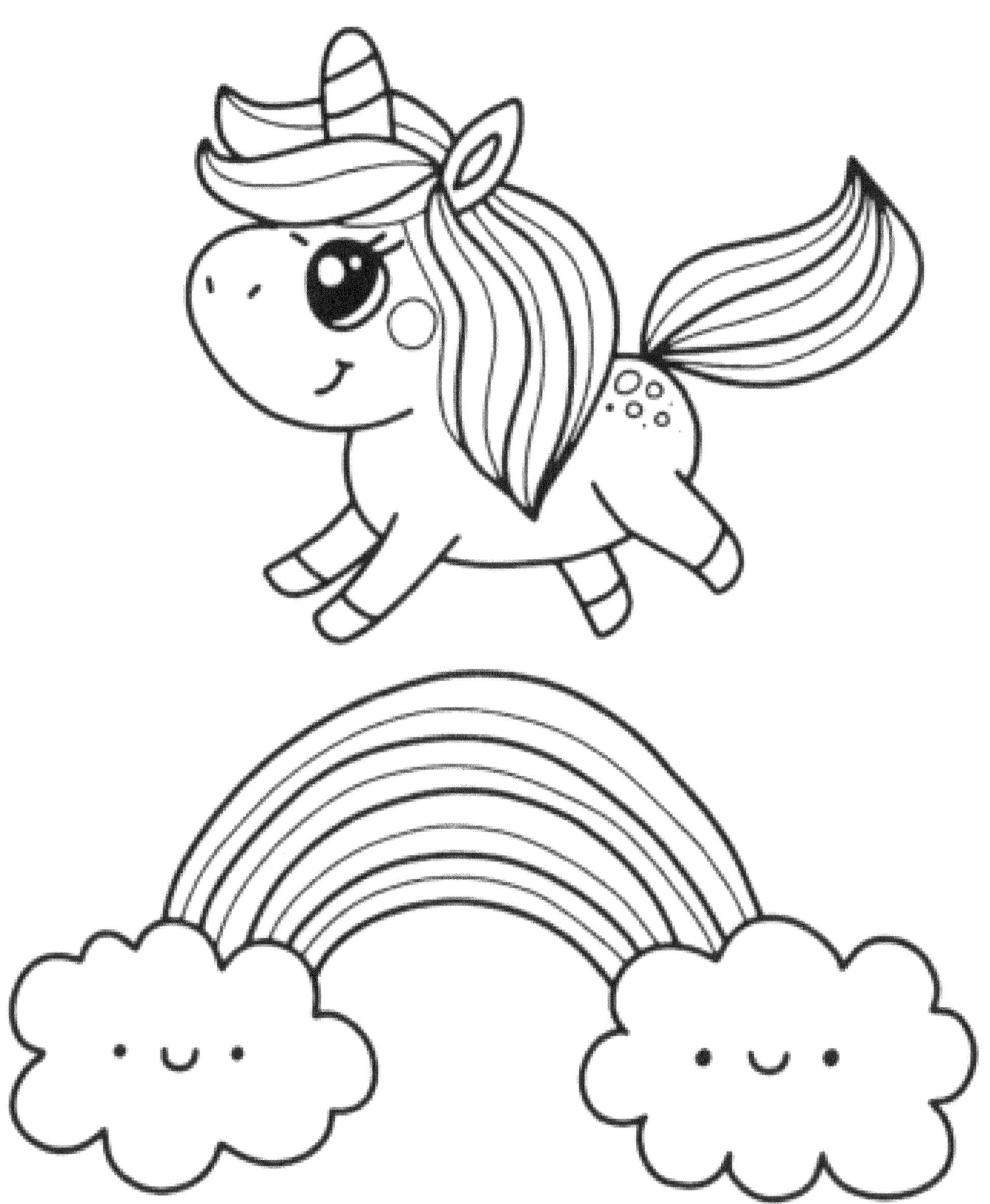

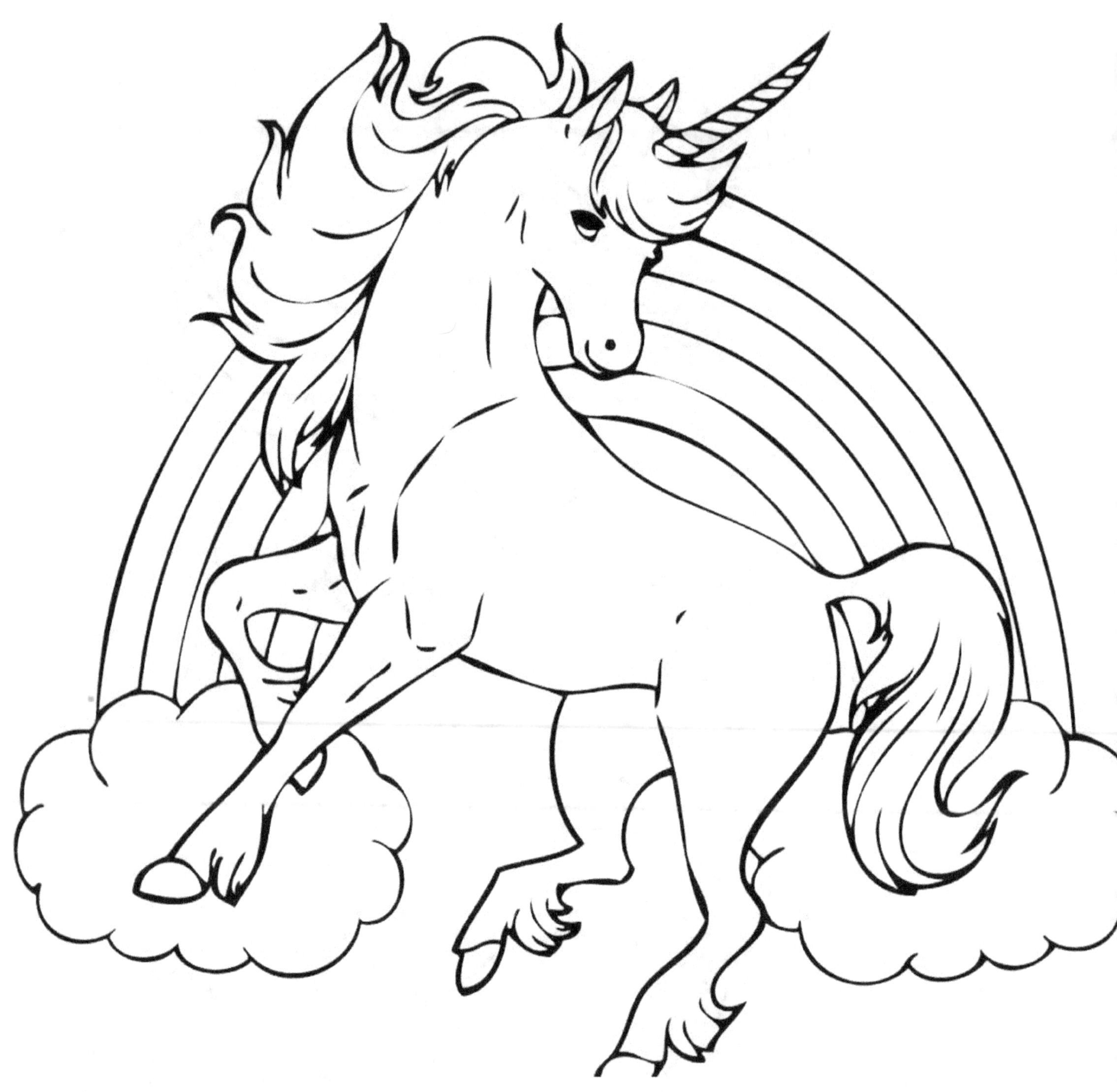

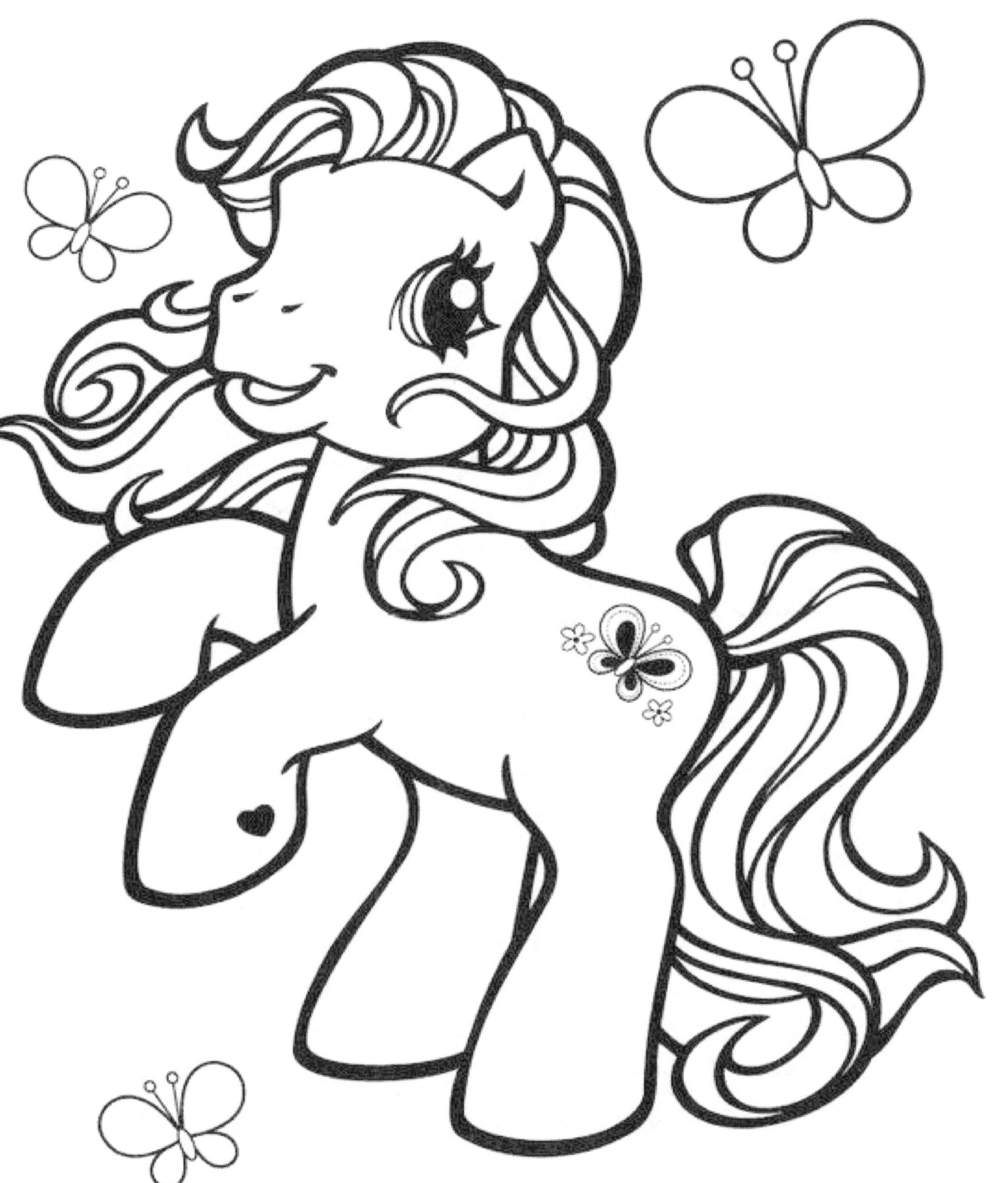

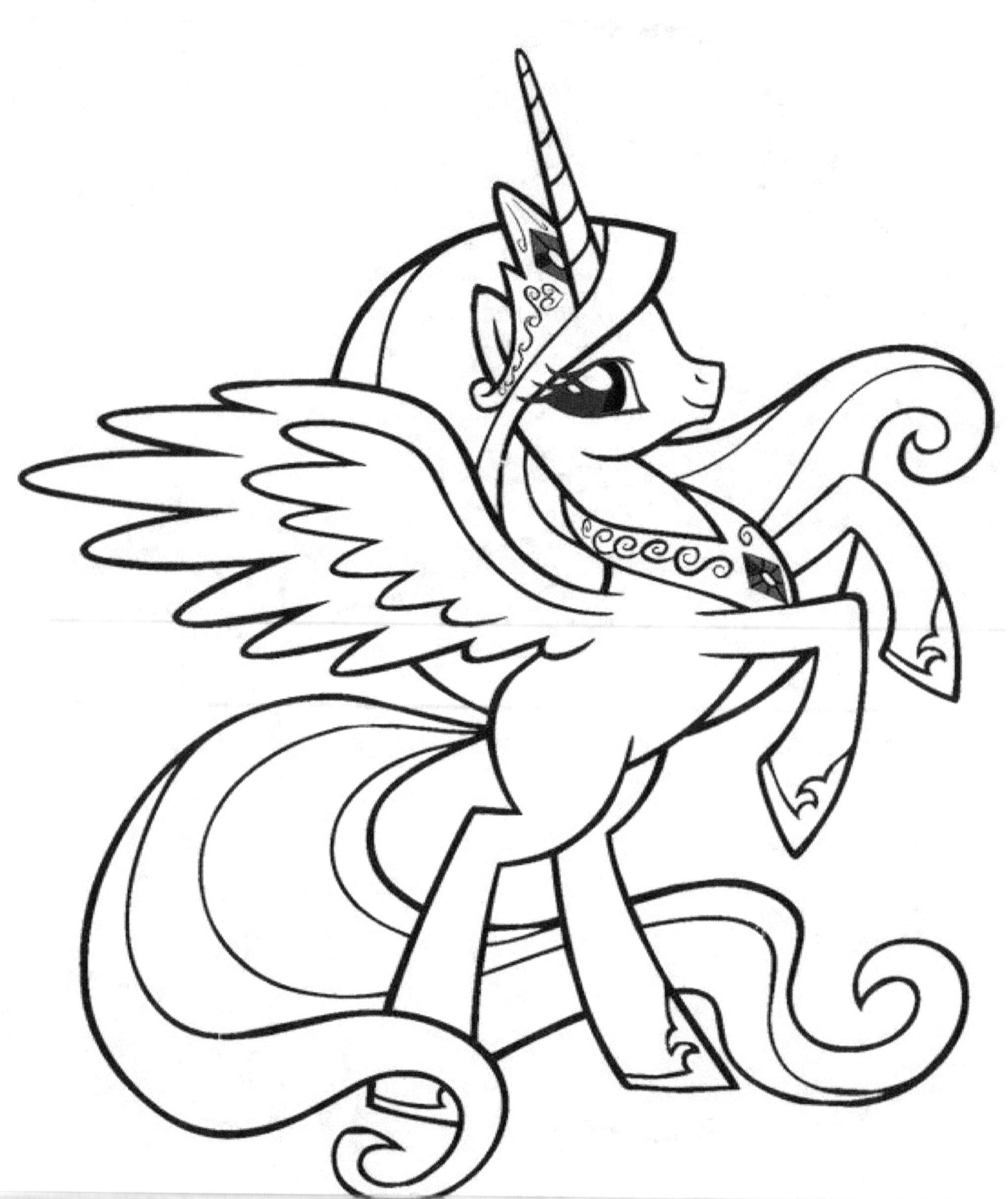

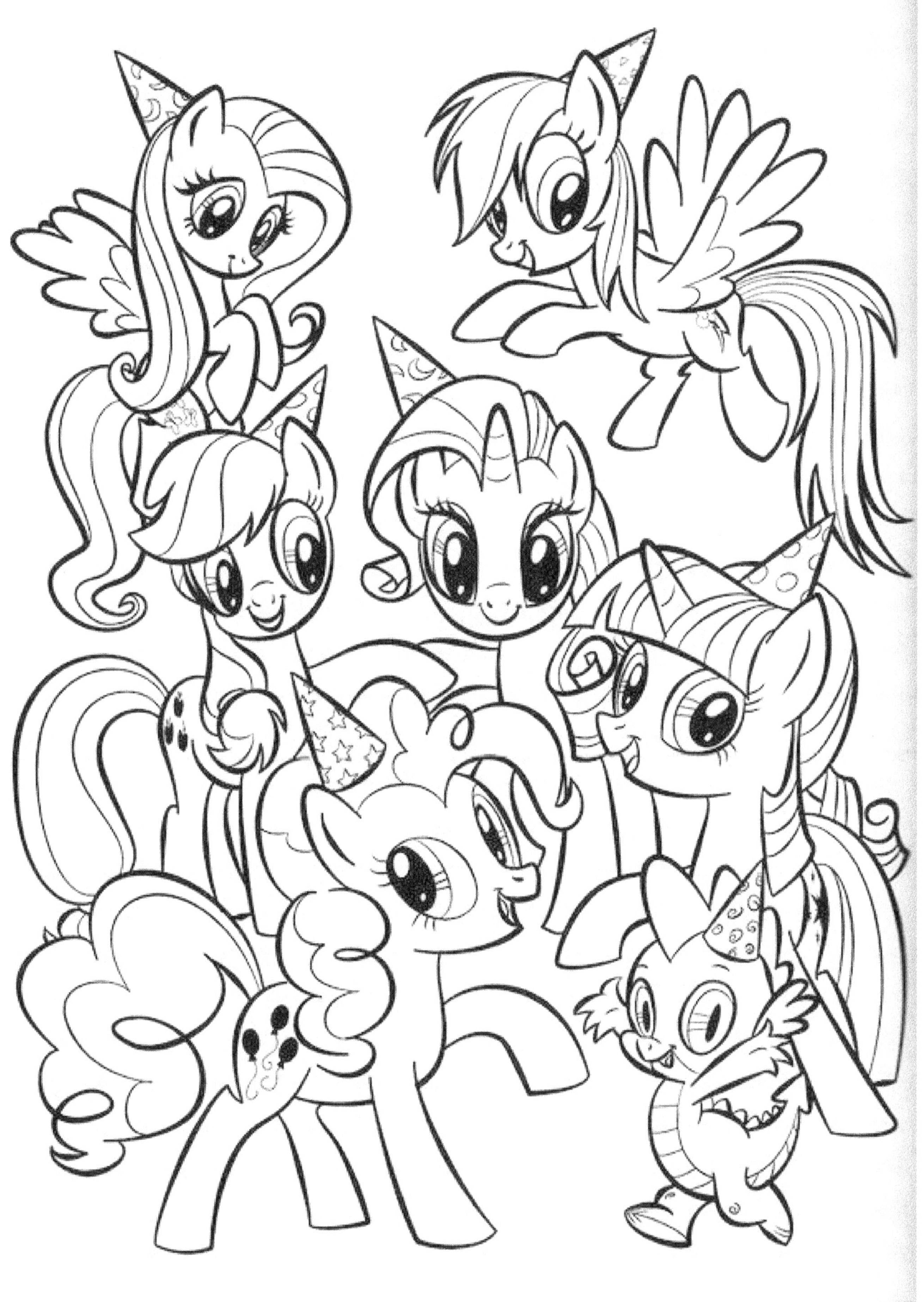

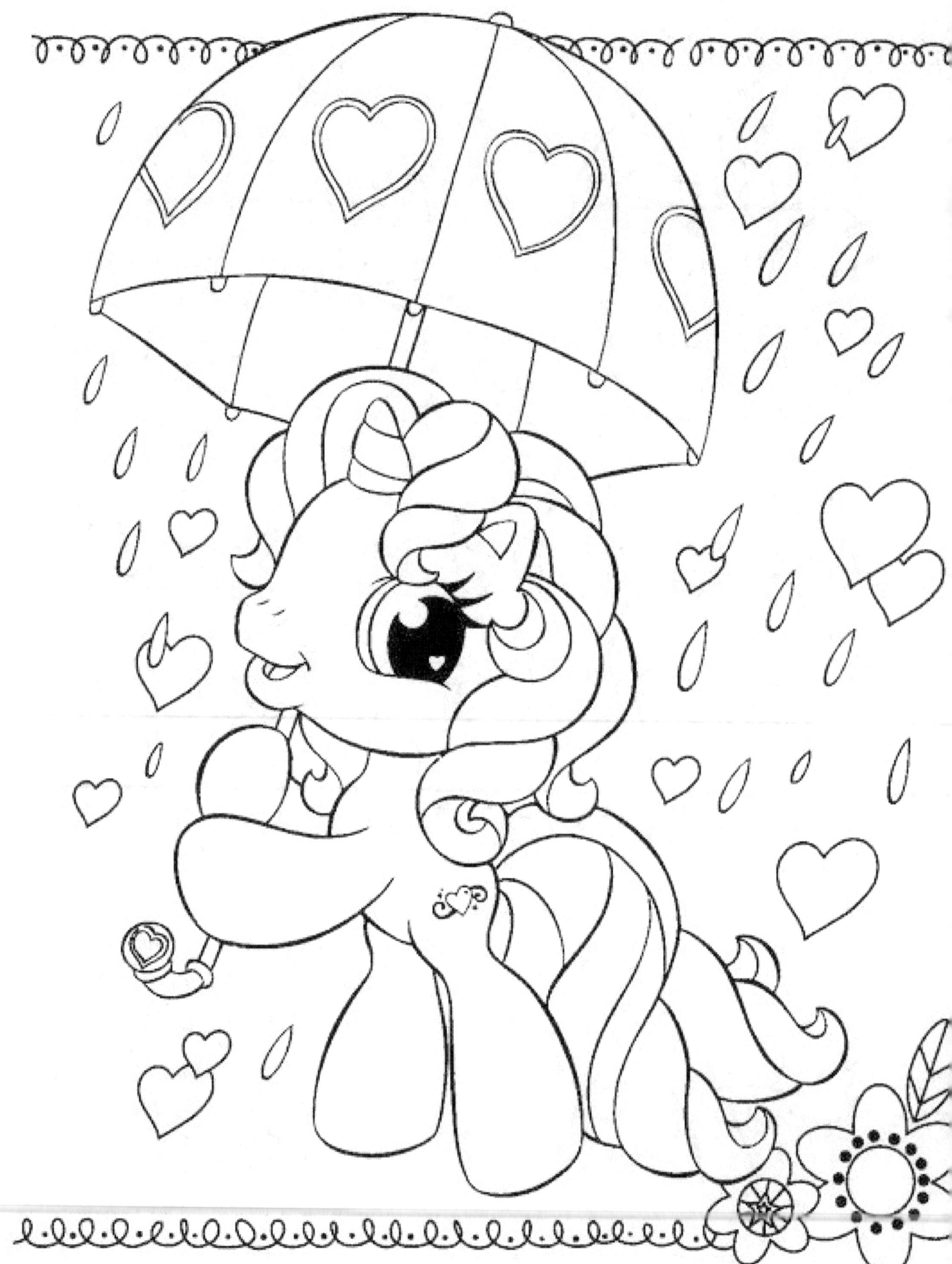